Action Research for Nurses

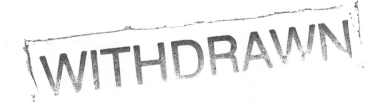

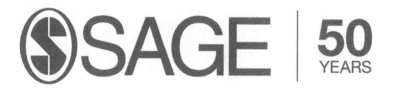

Action Research for Nurses

Peter McDonnell
Jean McNiff

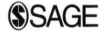

Los Angeles | London | New Delhi
Singapore | Washington DC

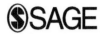

Los Angeles | London | New Delhi
Singapore | Washington DC

SAGE Publications Ltd
1 Oliver's Yard
55 City Road
London EC1Y 1SP

SAGE Publications Inc.
2455 Teller Road
Thousand Oaks, California 91320

SAGE Publications India Pvt Ltd
B 1/I 1 Mohan Cooperative Industrial Area
Mathura Road
New Delhi 110 044

SAGE Publications Asia-Pacific Pte Ltd
3 Church Street
#10-04 Samsung Hub
Singapore 049483

Editor: Mila Steele
Assistant editor: James Piper
Production editor: Katie Forsythe
Copyeditor: Rosemary Campbell
Marketing manager: Camille Richmond
Cover design: Shaun Mercier
Typeset by: C&M Digitals (P) Ltd, Chennai, India
Printed and bound by CPI Group (UK) Ltd,
Croydon, CR0 4YY

Library of Congress Control Number: 2015939590

British Library Cataloguing in Publication data

A catalogue record for this book is available from
the British Library

MIX
Paper from
responsible sources
FSC
www.fsc.org   FSC® C013604

ISBN 978-1-4739-1939-6
ISBN 978-1-4739-1940-2 (pbk)

Contents

List of figures and tables

FIGURES

TABLES

About the authors

Peter McDonnell has been a registered nurse since the 1970s and has a Masters degree in practitioner educational research. He has worked in both general and psychiatric nursing, and has extensive experience in healthcare management. You can contact Peter at mcdonnell.peter@outlook.com.

Jean McNiff is Professor of Educational Research at York St John University, and holds other international appointments as Visiting Professor. She works with practitioners in a range of settings. Jean writes books and other resources on action research across the professions, and her work is used globally on higher education and professional development courses. You can contact Jean at jeanmcniff@mac.com.

Acknowledgements

We wish to thank the editorial staff at Sage Publications who have been unfailingly helpful and supportive. We especially wish to thank Katie Metzler for her faith in the original idea.

Thank you also to Margaret, Julian, Tracy, David, Henry, Joseph and Reggie.

Introduction

This book is about doing action research in nursing contexts. It is written for practising clinical nurses, nursing students, nurse educators and nurse managers. It is also designed as a resource for nurses studying on postgraduate courses and for those seeking to continue their ongoing professional development and thereby improve their practices. The book offers ideas about how and why practices should be improved and how this may be done most effectively.

A key premise that runs through the book is that what people do is informed by what they know: how you speak is informed by your knowledge of language and context; how you write depends on whether you know how to write and are confident about your subject matter. It is the same with nursing: the practice of nursing is informed by what nurses know.

Three basic questions therefore arise:

- What constitutes nursing knowledge?
- How is nursing knowledge acquired?
- How is nursing knowledge put to use? (see also Chomsky, 1986: 3)

Most textbooks about nursing practice and education address these questions, though most do so from a conventional didactic perspective. They explain what nurses need to know about nursing as a topic (Peate and Nair, 2011; Reid-Searl et al., 2012), and what they need to do in practice (Benner et al., 2010; Higgs and Titchen, 2001). Current responses to the question usually show a commitment to scientific ways of thinking. There is an underpinning assumption that 'received technical rational knowledge' is correct, and nurses simply need to learn and apply this knowledge to their practices. Nurses should consult a book or a senior colleague to know how to check a blood pressure reading or change an infusion bag. These days, also, there is an increasing expectation that nurses will know how to handle technology and how to write prescriptions.

However, while acknowledging the importance of these approaches, this book takes a different view that is firmly rooted in practice, and that places the patient at the centre of the enquiry. We maintain that:

- nursing is about caring and ensuring the wellbeing of patients up to the point of outcome, whether recovery or death;
- nurses bring a good deal of wisdom to their practices, much of it tacit and acquired through experience, supplemented by ideas gained from textbooks and more experienced colleagues;
- nurses use their knowledge to ensure their practices are the best they can be for the benefit of their patients, their families, and for themselves.

Therefore, as well as asking more abstract questions about what nursing is and what nursing as a profession aims to do, we also raise practical questions about what nurses know and need to know about their own practices, how they acquire this knowledge and how they use it. It is not so much what other people know about nursing practices as what nurses know themselves and how they can improve their knowledge and therefore their practices. This means you. It also means that nursing may be seen as an educational practice, where nurses learn with and from patients and colleagues, and enable them to do the same. Patients are seen as people with considerable powers of discernment, able to make choices about their own wellbeing. It is the job of nurses to encourage these capacities and to learn with and from the patients they care for. The way to do this is through dialogue. These matters are discussed throughout the book.

These questions have become increasingly important in recent times, because nursing is currently at an all-time critical point, as explained in some detail in Chapter 2. Nurses are under fire from many directions and are regularly blamed for systemic failures, many of which have led to the deaths of patients. Reports such as the Francis (2013) and Berwick (2013) Reports attest to this. However, this blame game is deeply unfair, because, albeit with some exceptions, it is not nurses themselves that are at fault so much as the system in which nurses are caught, a system that systematically moves them away from the patients who represent the reasons for their hopes of taking up nursing as a caring profession. This book aims to give nurses the intellectual, practical and political resources to challenge and change the situation, and to take control of and reclaim their own professionalism. We argue that all nurses have considerable practical professional knowledge, that they can contribute to knowledge of the profession, and can shape and influence policy debates about the nature of nursing and the directions it should take.

At this point therefore we introduce one of the main contextualising frameworks of the book, that of the politics of knowledge. Political struggles can be seen across all knowledge domains – social, historical, organisational – and across all disciplines and professions, including nursing. These are always to do with what counts as valid knowledge, who counts as a valid knower, and who makes valid decisions about these things. Two such domains are especially important for nursing: (1) the politics of nursing knowledge and how this informs nursing practices; and (2) the politics of research knowledge and how this informs research practices. The two are parallel and mutually interdependent.

First we consider debates about the politics of nursing knowledge, and how this informs nursing practices.

THE POLITICS OF NURSING KNOWLEDGE

There is intense debate about what nursing knowledge is, whose knowledge is publicly accepted as legitimate, and who says so. Also, given as we said earlier that knowledge informs practices, the debates extend to who owns nursing practices, with far-reaching implications that if you own the knowledge you own the practice, and therefore, ultimately, the profession.

The current owners of nursing knowledge, and therefore of the practice and the profession are mainly nurses in senior administrative, non-clinical practice-based positions in professional bodies and universities, acting largely on behalf of statutory professional authorities. In Chapter 2 we tell the story of how this situation has come about. It is these elites who represent nurses in general. Each group has its own agenda, usually to promote a specific image of nursing as a profession, which is communicated through the mainstream media and political rhetoric. The increasingly generic view presented is that nursing is an abstract, high-tech, high-ticket, intellectually-oriented discipline whose main stock in trade is the conventional form of theory of nursing practices. Anyone wishing to become a nurse must first go into higher education to learn the theory, which they will be expected later to apply to practice. This is bad news for anyone who does not achieve appropriate school-leaving grades, which will disbar them from entry, as we discuss later. The everyday practices of care, in many contexts, are not legitimate topics of discourse, though, following Francis, there has recently been a massive surge in the official rhetoric about the need for care and patient-centred nursing (see, among others, websites for the Patient-Centred Care Resource Centre, the National Institute for Health and Care Excellence (NICE) and the Royal College of Nursing (RCN)). This rhetoric is somewhat contradicted in practice by the fact that everyday clinical area caring practices are still allocated largely to unqualified healthcare assistants. Textbook knowledge takes precedence over the everyday knowledge of people and their lifeworlds.

While this leaning towards abstract theory and disciplines-based rhetoric may be fine for people such as barristers who by definition ply a talking trade, it is no good for patients or nurses, given that nursing and caring for patients is a hands-on practice. No one should be surprised at the increased incidences of bedsores and dehydration reported in the Francis Report, given that the nursing students who are learning to prevent such things are daily sequestered in lecture halls where such topics are dealt with from a theoretical perspective rather than as a real-world experience.

To help appreciate the ironies of this situation, consider this analogy by Donald Schön. In his seminal *The Reflective Practitioner* (1983) and in later work (1995), Schön wrote about the topology of professional landscapes. He said there was a high hard ground, populated mainly by established academics who produced a conventional, scientific kind of knowledge by doing 'pure' research. The value of the research was acknowledged by themselves and by those who used its findings, and all agreed that this knowledge would contribute to good theory. Down below the high ground were some swampy lowlands (Schön's words), populated by ordinary people who produced practical, everyday knowledge. This kind of knowledge, however, was not seen as the right kind that would count as or contribute to theory, so it continued to be called practical knowledge. Everyone, both on the high ground and in the swampy lowlands, agreed with the situation, with how different people were positioned and how their different kinds of knowledge were allocated different kinds of status. The irony for Schön was that the knowledge and theory produced on the high ground was used by a limited number of people, often for their own self or professional promotion as academics, whereas the everyday practical knowledge of those in the swampy lowlands was the kind of knowledge that kept the world turning but was not seen as high-stakes knowledge or valid theory.

The nursing profession, as represented by official professional bodies and by nurse academics seems to have bought into this same epistemological hierarchy, where technical rational knowledge – 'know that' – is seen as the best kind, and practical skills-based or embodied knowledge as less than the best. Narrow judgements are made about the quality of knowledge and the research that produces it by means of statistical data and analysis. It is the case that we measure that which can be measured instead of appreciating that other kinds of knowledge exist that may more effectively communicate the real-life everyday experiences that make up most clinical nurses' and patients' lives. The body of knowledge that develops from this reductionist view of research is then taught to nursing students, who are selected for entry to the profession through the narrow portal identified above that accepts academic qualifications relating only to this kind of knowledge. Thus the system perpetuates itself and provides its own legitimating structures. The net effect is that new students enter the profession through this narrow portal while thousands of experienced nurses leave by the back door, often because they see their daily work as undervalued and unrepresented by the elites who set the course for the profession.

Schön's ideas are still relevant today across the professions, although in many places the topology is beginning to level out, supported by new directions towards a new form of knowledge base in the professions. Eraut (1994), for example, speaks about the need to recognise the contributions of different kinds of professional knowledge and different modes of knowledge production, a theme also developed in the work of, for example, Gibbons et al. (1994) who emphasise the need for practice-based forms of knowledge and knowledge production. This view is also promoted by researchers such as Sternberg and Horvath (1999) who, drawing on work by philosophers such as Polanyi (1958, 1983), highlight the importance of the tacit dimension in professional practice, and by Taylor (2000), Winter and Munn-Giddings (2001) and Ghaye and Lillyman (2010) on the importance of personal self-reflection in health and social care. Interestingly, precisely these attributes are recommended by the Francis Report (2013) as possible contributions to remedying the present-day cultures of bullying, high-handed managerialism and misplaced, misdirected care.

However, in nursing the existing topology is still firmly entrenched, influenced strongly by its history and its current representation in the literatures. The situation will change only if clinical nurses within the profession decide to change it. It is their profession and only they can negotiate how they wish it to develop, in whose interests it should change, and how this might happen. This means, as Arendt (1958) says, exercising one's agency from an understanding that collaborative focused action can have political impact. This is where action research comes in. Yet it is also where the politics of research knowledge comes in.

THE POLITICS OF RESEARCH KNOWLEDGE

The dominant form of research that generates the dominant form of knowledge is as outlined by Schön above. Technical rational forms of scientific or social scientific research generate technical rational forms of knowledge, which is the basis of abstract conceptual forms of theory. Further, the hierarchisation of research and its knowledge outputs is reflected, as in nursing, in the social structures of the research community. Also as in nursing, the issue of what counts as research and who can do it is deeply contested. It is assumed that only those who are officially recognised as researchers are qualified to do real research.

There is a deep ironic contradiction here. These days the language of research is everywhere in nursing practices and nurse education. While it is not yet compulsory for clinical nurses to do research (i.e. be research active), there is a clear expectation that they should be at least 'research literate' or 'research aware' (Moule and Hek, 2011: 1–12), that is, have a working knowledge of what research means and how it is done. Further, while research may not yet be compulsory for all nurses, continuing professional development is. Research is an essential part of this and research means learning. Research is also compulsory for those nurses who wish to pursue higher degree accreditation, even at bachelor's level. Further, following the introduction of evidence-based practice within medicine in the 1990s, the nursing profession has been quick to adopt the same philosophy and terminology, and there are now calls for nurses to produce evidence on a regular basis to show that they are competent and able both as clinical practitioners and as researchers (Moule and Hek, 2011).

Amidst all this grand rhetoric, however, there are few calls for a demonstration of a critical understanding of what the rhetoric means. What do 'research' and 'evidence-based practice' mean, given that there are many kinds of research and many kinds of evidence, generated from many kinds of data? What does it mean to be a researcher?

Most mainstream textbooks would respond according to the standard doctrine, that doing research in nursing is about knowing the literatures and applying established theories to your practices (Melnyk and Fineout-Overholt, 2005). The standard doctrine also states that qualified researchers (people in higher education or official offices) should do research while nurses should take the role of research participants, possibly to gather data which they then supply to the real researchers, or even becoming data in real researchers' research. This can lead to what Eikeland (2011) calls a system of 'condescending ethics', part of an 'othering business', where official researchers give a passing nod to issues of inclusion but continue to include others on their own officially established terms. It is easy to talk about participation but it is questionable who participates, how they participate and what role they serve.

We take a different view. We believe that, instead of only consuming officially sanctioned research, all practising clinical nurses should do research, not necessarily of the conventional scientific statistics-oriented variety, but as a form of everyday practice where they ask questions of the kind, 'How do I investigate and make sense of what I am doing? How do I improve it?' This requires nurses to research their everyday practices in action, and to be able to explain to others, including patients, colleagues, families and friends, what they are doing and why they are doing it. This kind of research is called action research, a form of enquiry that is well established in other disciplines and is now actively visible in nursing, albeit (with some notable exceptions) still at an abstract textbook level, and that now needs a new body of practical knowledge, provided by nurses for nurses, to show its power for shaping the future of the profession.

To achieve this, the book proposes that nurses use an action research approach to investigate their practices as reflective practitioners, recognising that they work in complex situations with daily challenges, where the needs of each patient represent unique demands. Unlike many other professions, much nurse development becomes out of date within months as technological innovations and scientific discoveries appear. Nursing is a vibrant, dynamic activity where every interaction brings new learning opportunities, thus challenging the concept of a static system of education. It is essential that nurses see the need to develop their own area of practice by deepening their understanding of what they are doing through researching their practices. The aim of the book therefore is to help them appreciate that developing themselves as researchers is perfectly achievable and beneficial, and to see the wider implications of their studies for education and new educational forms of nursing theory.

This view is of course not welcome in many places, because, as noted, nursing as a profession is underpinned by a specific knowledge base produced by the bureaucratic and academic elites spoken of above. The knowledge that comprises the knowledge base tends to take the form of academic scientific knowledge; the everyday practical knowledge of nurses is not seen as valid or worthy of inclusion, and the caring values base that is at the heart of clinical nursing is factored out. Unfortunately, the situation remains that, to challenge the dominance of the established form, both of the knowledge and of the system that maintains its dominance, is to say goodbye to nursing as a career, because, as noted, you can be accepted as a nurse only by demonstrating that you are knowledgeable about the accepted form of knowledge, which means you have to buy into the system. Given that these days nursing contracts carry certain gagging orders that prevent you speaking about professional conditions, you are either stuck in an oppressive, self-congratulatory system or you can choose to leave. Which is what countless promising nurses do (see, for example, comments from 2013 editions of the *Health Service Journal* at www.hsj.co.uk/news/thousands-of-nurses-exit-the-profession/5065729.article; the *Nursing Times* article at www.nursingtimes.net/nursing-practice/specialisms/management/exclusive-numbers-choosing-to-leave-nursing-rise-by-26/5065685. article; and a 2014 analysis from *The Nursing Standard* at http://rcnpublishing. com/doi/pdfplus/10.7748/ns.29.2.14.s19).

This situation is wrong. It is wrong for patients and wrong for nurses, as explained in Chapter 2. It is also wrong for the profession, because any system that continues to focus inwards from a self-serving perspective is unsustainable and will eventually implode, which is what nursing is doing at the moment. Nursing needs to develop a new focus that has the interests of the patient at its heart, as recommended by the Francis Report (2013) and The King's Fund (2013) report *Patient-Centred Leadership: Rediscovering Our Purpose*, and this can come about only if nurses themselves see the need for action – both epistemological action, which is about knowledge, and communicative action: nurses need to see themselves as able and competent knowers of their own practices and be prepared to say this. But to do this, they need to engage in research, of a kind that will help them to make sense of what they are doing with a view to creating a new knowledge base for the profession, produced by nurses for nurses. This both places research in the areas where practice is carried out and it also turns everyday practice into research activity.

Nurses need to develop confidence that they are able to do research. We emphasise that research is not the preserve only of academics but can be undertaken by anyone. The book aims to help you see how you can do research too, and takes you through the process whereby you research your own practice and learn from the experience. It gives advice about how you do it, why you need to do it, and how you can use your knowledge to create a more equitable and compassionate profession that includes all and serves the interests of all.

This does mean choices, but the benefits are potentially amazingly far-reaching, for individual nurses, for patients and for healthcare services in general.

A NOTE ABOUT THE RESEARCH BASE FOR THIS BOOK

This book is grounded in the real-life accounts of practising nurses with whom we have worked directly over the years in different countries and clinical settings. The stories presented as examples in the text are drawn from interviews conducted with them, and are published with their approval and permission.

I

WHAT IS ACTION RESEARCH? WHY IS IT RELEVANT FOR NURSES?

This part deals with the questions, 'What is action research? Why is it relevant for nurses?' It outlines ideas about what you need to know about action research, why you need to know it and its relevance for your practice as a nurse, and some of the ethical issues involved. It touches on the philosophy and history of nursing and of action research.

The part contains Chapters 1, 2 and 3.

CHAPTER 1 WHAT DO YOU NEED TO KNOW ABOUT ACTION RESEARCH?

This chapter asks the question, 'What do you need to know about action research?' It considers what is involved in all kinds of research, followed by descriptions of how action research is distinctive, how you do it, and some of its core assumptions. Purposes and aims of action research are identified. The chapter outlines ideas about knowledge claims, researcher positionality, the differences between professional development and action research, and the values-oriented nature of action research. It also explains how action research can take the form of social and political activism.

CHAPTER 2 WHY SHOULD NURSES DO ACTION RESEARCH?

This chapter asks, 'Why should nurses do action research?' It discusses issues of epistemology, theory and logic, as well as the idea of shifting paradigms. A brief history of the historical changes in the structures, focus and delivery of nurse education is outlined. The chapter also contains suggestions about why nurses should do action research from the perspective of perceiving oneself as a competent theorist as well as a capable practitioner. This involves exercising the right to research, which brings with it responsibilities to research. By doing action research, nurses can contribute to a new scholarship of teaching and learning for nursing.

CHAPTER 3   ETHICAL ISSUES

This chapter outlines issues regarding ethical guidelines in nursing and in educational research. Some questions are raised regarding the value of guidelines like these, as well as some contradictions internal to the guidelines. Two important conceptual frameworks are offered: system and lifeworld and knowledge-constituted interests. A further important concept of researcher positionality is discussed. The chapter considers an ethics of action research for nursing.

ONE

What do you need to know about action research?

This chapter is about what action research is and what it means for nurses to do it. The chapter asks questions such as:

- What do you need to know about action research? Why do you need to know it?
- How do you do action research?
- What are the core assumptions of action research?

Briefly, action research is a form of enquiry that helps you as a nurse find ways to evaluate and improve your practice where necessary. You learn how to do things differently, which means that you create new knowledge about what you are doing. Doing action research also enables you to communicate this new knowledge to others so that they can learn from you how they might do the same. Potentially you can contribute to other people's learning and thereby to the development of your profession. Action research is therefore by nature educational.

To appreciate what action research involves and how to do it means first appreciating what is involved in doing all kinds of research. This chapter is organised to address the following questions:

1. What is involved in all kinds of research?
2. What do you need to know specifically about action research? Why do you need to know it?
3. What are the core assumptions of action research?
4. What are the purposes and uses of action research?

Chapter 2 develops these ideas by asking why it is important for nurses to do action research, how the knowledge generated may be used, and some of the choices involved.

First, then, consider what is involved in all kinds of research.

1. WHAT IS INVOLVED IN ALL KINDS OF RESEARCH?

All research, including action research, involves the following:

- Doing research enables you to make a claim to knowledge. You test the validity (truthfulness, believability) of the claim through gathering data and generating evidence, with a view to contributing to new theory.
- The research contains a philosophical base, which gives you explanations for the research and its methodology. You can state the reasons and purposes for doing it, and for doing it in a particular way.
- The research has a practical element, which contains advice about the methodological steps involved in order to achieve its reasons and purposes.
- The research contains a written element, which serves to communicate the research findings.
- The research requires critical reflection, which enables you to articulate the significance of what you have done and found, and what needs to be done next.

Doing research enables you to make a claim to knowledge

Research is always about knowledge, whether this means discovering knowledge and finding things out that you did not know before (the knowledge is new for you), or creating original knowledge that no one knew before (the knowledge is new for everyone). As a nurse you can contribute to existing knowledge of the field; this could be in the general field of nursing, or in a specialised field such as psychiatric nursing or children's nursing.

If you wish to make a knowledge claim (you claim that something is known now that was not known before, whether by you or someone else), you need to test its validity, that is, to demonstrate its truthfulness or believability. Testing and demonstrating the validity of knowledge claims therefore comes to stand as a sign of researcher authenticity and responsibility. When you write your dissertation or report, virtually the entire text is given over to testing and demonstrating the validity of your knowledge claim. How you do this is explained in Chapter 7.

The knowledge you create can contribute to new theory. Broadly speaking, the word 'theory' means 'explanation'. You can say, 'I have a theory about [I think I can explain] how and why we can help psychiatric patients be more involved in their own wellbeing'. We all have millions of theories like this that guide our everyday practices. When you actively research your practices and come up with innovative ideas about how to involve psychiatric patients in their own wellbeing and why you should do so, you can claim two things:

1. You can claim these ideas as new knowledge, and say, 'I have developed strategies for engaging psychiatric patients in their own wellbeing'.
2. You can also claim that you have generated a theory of practice: this means you can explain how and why you have developed new strategies. When you generate theory, you outline the reasons and purposes for what you are doing, explain how this is grounded in appropriate research procedures, and show how the validity of your emergent knowledge claims has been tested against the stringent critique of peers and others.

Consider these knowledge claims:

- [I know that] Mr Green is recovering well.
- I have studied counselling and developed my therapeutic skills.
- I know the importance of reflective practice in nursing.

Each claim implies that you know what you know and you know how you have come to know it.

To get to this point of articulating claims to knowledge and the processes that have led up to them, it is useful to be able to use some specific terminology, especially the words 'ontology, 'epistemology' and 'methodology'.

Ontology refers to a theory of being, how you view yourself. Your ontological values are to do with matters of identity and inform who you think you are.

Epistemology refers to a theory of knowledge, a theory of knowledge acquisition and creation, and a theory of testing the validity of knowledge claims: in other words, you are able to say what you know and how you have come to know it, and explain how you have checked that what you say may be believed.

Methodology refers to how we do things. It is different from 'methods', which refers to specific techniques such as when gathering or analysing data.

The research contains a philosophical base, which gives you explanations for the research and its methodology

Research is never undertaken in a vacuum: you need to give reasons for doing it (say why the research is necessary) and your purposes (say what you hope to achieve). Research therefore becomes political, because it aims to destabilise and possibly change established personal, social and institutional structures through developing new thinking and practices. This carries implications for researchers, because it then becomes their responsibility always to interrogate contexts that are otherwise taken for granted. Several major authors speak about the need for critique. Hannah Arendt uses the analogy of a pearl diver 'who descends to the bottom of the sea … to pry loose the rich and the strange, the pearls and the coral in the depths and to carry them to the surface …' (Arendt, 1968: 205). Foucault constantly emphasises the need to 'make the familiar strange' (e.g. Foucault, 1980a).

Interrogating contexts helps us to become aware of what is going on, and of our own social, political and historical situatedness, that is, our involvement in the situation we are investigating. We tend usually to take these things for granted without questioning them. Bourdieu (1990) uses the analogy that a fish does not know it is in water. By doing research we can make ourselves aware that we are in water, and of the state of the water we are in and where it comes from. We especially become aware of how we learn to accept what is said and not to inter-rogate the language used to communicate messages. These matters are especially meaningful for nursing. Rolfe (1996, 1998), for example, tells the story of how, historically, nursing has been positioned as subservient to medicine; how nurses' knowledge still remains subjugated; and how many members of the establish-ment still refuse to accept nurses' theories of practice as serious contributions to the field. It is the same issue outlined by al-Takriti (2010), who speaks about 'negligent mnemocide', when colonised people's collective memories are eradi-cated through the imposition of the coloniser's language and traditions. Many of the nurses we spoke with in our research appeared to feel something similar: many felt that a huge part of their own knowledge base had been erased because it does not fit into the currently accepted models. Perhaps, instead of discounting those aspects for which we have no language to describe or means to measure, we should develop a new language by carrying out research into our own work areas that is more relevant and fit for purpose than the accepted dominant form.

The research has a practical element, which contains advice about the practical steps involved in order to achieve its goals and purposes

All research is, in Stenhouse's (1983) words, 'systematic enquiry made public'. Action research has the additional element of contributing to social transforma-tion towards democratic and egalitarian ways of being (McNiff, 2013).

However, there are different kinds of research, each with their own method-ologies, forms and methods. Conventional social science research, which is the basis for most nurse research, tends to adopt a linear format. It begins with a hypothesis and follows a straight path towards a final answer: a → b → c → d → the end, aiming to show the cause and effect relationship of 'If x, then y'. Action research, on the other hand, is generally understood to follow a cyclical process of plan → act → observe → reflect → re-plan … though there are many variations on the theme (see Figure 1.1).

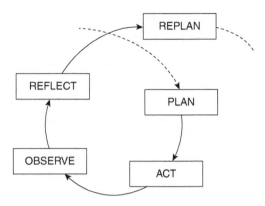

Figure 1.1 The cyclical nature of action research

The metaphors of action research are those of emergent processes with mutual reciprocal influence, where the whole contains multiple interrelated parts and each part contains the whole within itself (see for example, Sumara and Davis, 2009). This complex systems perspective is different from a reductionist perspective that

> ... generates knowledge and understanding of phenomena by breaking them down into constituent parts and then studying these simple elements in terms of cause and effect. With systems thinking the belief is that the world is systemic, which means that phenomena are understood to be an emergent property of an interrelated whole. *Emergence* and *interrelatedness* are the fundamental ideas of systems thinking. (Flood, 2001: 133, emphasis in original)

These ideas about emergence and interrelatedness are especially relevant to nursing, which is about helping others to move back into wellbeing and maintain their sense of coherence as a whole person. Nursing itself has moved beyond the curative and preventative models of the 1990s towards a twenty-first-century relational view, which we develop in this book as a dialogical model. The ideas are also important because they show the theoretical commensurability between the philosophy and methodology of action research and nursing. In action research researchers work collaboratively with one another, while in nursing the patient is not seen as a 'what' (a case or the recipient of a procedure: see also Liaschenko, 1997) but as a 'who', an active partner in a constellation of other agents and actors, a participant in a dialogue of equals. This has considerable implications for the ethics of nursing (Chapter 3) and the development of an educational, dialogical view of nursing.

The research contains a written element, which serves to communicate the research findings

Research of all kinds needs to be made public in order to communicate its findings and knowledge claims and its potential significance for different areas. Writing is not an add-on undertaken after the event but is a main vehicle for making sense of practices. It serves many purposes in research, including the production of reports, writing for a higher degree, and writing articles for publication in academic and peer-reviewed journals (Williamson et al., 2012: 170–187; see also Burnard et al., 2011).

Writing can also act as a form of reflective practice, a process of making explicit what is implicit. This is a core aspect of professional learning: Schön (1983, 1995), Eraut (1994) and Sternberg and Horvath (1999) all speak about the need to recognise professional competence as rooted in the tacit knowledge of the practitioner. Within a clinical nursing context, Higgs and Titchen (2001) emphasise that knowledge always belongs to a knower, and that professional craft knowledge is essential to nursing competence. Using the analogy of an iceberg, Titchen and Ersser (2001: 48) make the point that 'only the tip of the iceberg is available for critical, public scrutiny and for its acquisition by others in their development of expertise'.

Writing therefore can act both as a means to record events and articulate their significance as well as a means of reflection and analysis. The capacity to reflect on one's actions and thinking, and to reframe these in light of better understandings is the basis for improving one's understanding of personal practice and of reframing existing frames of understanding (Schön and Rein, 1994).

The research requires critical reflection, which enables you to articulate the significance of what you have done and found, and what needs to be done next

When we do research we always need to ask, 'So what? What is the point of doing it?' Sennett (2008) tells the story of how Hannah Arendt stopped him in the street to make sure he would communicate through his writing the fact that 'people who make things usually don't understand what they are doing' (p. 1). Research is a form of making, creating knowledge that did not exist before. But it can also be like Pandora's box, where evils are released as well as good things. When you do research be as clear as possible about what you are doing it for. The purpose of action research is always to influence processes of personal and social change. Check also that you are living in the direction of your values and not compromising them. This kind of conflict of values is illustrated by a comment from one of our research participants:

> I was offered the attractive opportunity to do research on two products and do a comparative analysis of them. I was told my research would benefit patients. However, on closer inspection I came to the conclusion that the two products were made by the same company, and any research report I produced would

have little benefit for the patients, and would mainly benefit the company. I decided against doing the research.

However, while reflection is essential in helping us to be clear about our reasons and purposes, reflection alone is insufficient to effect social change. Social change happens when people think about things and decide to take focused action. Mendieta reports Rorty's views that:

> When faced with opponents who don't share our worldview ... we cannot hope to refute them, but we can concretely elucidate our worldview in the hope that it will make their worldview look untenable. 'There is no answer to a redescription', [Rorty] pronounced, 'save a re-re-description'. (2006: 10–11)

Mendieta terms this 'incremental redescription', which is what often happens in action research: we take action, reflect, re-act, re-reflect, and so on, in a never ending incremental flow of expanding action and reflection.

Now consider what is involved specifically in action research.

2. WHAT DO YOU NEED TO KNOW SPECIFICALLY ABOUT ACTION RESEARCH? WHY DO YOU NEED TO KNOW IT?

This section addresses the following issues:

1. What action research is and what it is not.
2. How do you do action research?

What action research is and what it is not

First, consider what action research is.

What action research is

Action research is a form of enquiry that enables practitioners in every job and in every walk of life to evaluate what they are doing and to find ways of doing it better. They look at their practice and the contexts they are in and ask, 'What am I doing? Is it satisfactory? If not, why not?' This helps them to take stock of and evaluate what they are doing. They also ask, 'What can I do to improve my practice? Why should I do this?' This helps them to take control of their practice and find ways of improving it as they see fit. They then systematically investigate it with the aim of describing and explaining what they are doing to other people and why they are doing it. The descriptions and explanations they give come to act as their personal professional theories of practice, which they can then share with others, and from which others may learn if they wish. When nurses improve their personal and collective knowledge of their practices they can use this knowledge to enhance the quality of their professionalism, as well as contribute to its enhancement and democratisation. Importantly they are able to identify patient needs, extend their practices out to their patients, and explain what they are doing and why they are doing it. Action research questions often take the form, 'How do I ...?' or 'How do we ...?' In this case nurses could develop individual or group research programmes around the questions:

- How do I help patients to take more informed control of their own medication? This will lead to greater independence and earlier identification of possible side effects.
- How can we teach new staff the essentials of oxygen administration and develop awareness of individual patients' requirements and responses?

What action research is not

Action research is not conventional scientific or social scientific research; action research and social science traditions are different in core respects of intent and methodology.

The aim of scientific research is to predict and control what will happen through demonstrating a cause and effect relationship between variables. You can test the effect of a drug on patient recovery through randomised controlled trials. A lot of nursing research takes the form of social science research and is based on the same assumptions and principles. It is assumed that you can influence a patient's progress through applying a specific procedure and monitoring the subsequent results. However, these approaches can be limited, mainly because they assume a simplistic cause and effect relationship. Real-world nursing is not like this. Patients are real people and need personalised care and comfort, much of which cannot be explained in terms of simplistic cause and effect relationships.

Social science perspectives permeate nurse education (Rolfe, 1998). It is assumed that nurses should learn a given body of knowledge and apply it to their practices. This often leads to what is called 'the theory-practice gap', that is, when well-formed 'pure' theory cannot be mapped onto untidy, frequently chaotic real-world practices. Sadly this assumption that theory can be directly applied to practice has often led to catastrophic practices, where nurses have focused so much on getting the application of theory right that the personal needs of patients have gone unnoticed. At least a positive outcome is that calls are now made for nurses to research their own practices and make their accounts public (see The King's Fund 2013 report). This means that nurses should do action research, which is premised on the idea that nurses (and all practitioners) can and should research their own practices.

These different research perspectives lead to different researcher position-alities. In social science forms, researchers stand outside a situation and ask, 'What are those people over there doing?' This kind of outsider research (also called 'spectator research') adopts an externalist, objectivist stance. Action research is usually insider research. Nurses see themselves as part of the con-text they are investigating and ask, 'Are we doing this right? How do we improve our work as necessary?' If they feel their work is reasonably satisfac-tory, they produce authenticated evidence to show why this may be the case. If they feel something needs improving, they work on that aspect, keeping records and producing regular oral and written progress reports about what they are doing.

Here are some examples of questions asked about nursing practices that show the difference between a social science outsider perspective and an action research insider perspective.

Examples of social science outsider questions are:

- What is the relationship between nurses' practice-based knowledge and the quality of patient care?
- What is the best way to apply a dressing?
- What is the effect of regular hydration practices on patients' wellbeing?

Examples of action research insider questions are:

- How do I improve my practices as a nurse for the benefit of patients?
- How do I learn to apply dressings?
- How do I ensure that patients get sufficient hydration?

Action research refers broadly to the processes involved in taking action for political action. The 'action' is always action in the world, with social and polit-ical intent: it aims to help others to live and think autonomously and enjoy full engagement with life. It means thinking carefully about what you hope to achieve, which means checking that what you intend to do will lead as much as possible to social good rather than to harm.

It is always important to remember that the term 'action research' contains two words – 'action' and 'research' – and that these refer to different things.

Action refers to what we do. There are different kinds of action: we can take unplanned action such as when we make a mistake in drug dosages. We can also take intentional, planned action, such as when we help patients get dressed. This is the kind of action that is relevant to action research.

Research refers to how we investigate and find out about what we do. We come to new understandings and create new knowledge. In action research the knowledge is always about practices, and involves investigating the reasons for, as well as the outcomes of, any actions we take.

> A high number of our patients have asthma, even though this may not be the primary cause of admission. I noticed that many do not seem to be making the best use of their inhalers because they use them at inappropriate times and not in the way they are intended for use. This concerns me because the long-term effects could be detrimental. I decided it would be a good idea to try to give updated advice on how they could best use them. I was aware that many people feel a great sense of ownership of their condition and can resent people interfering as they see it. I decided, as first step, to have a brief discussion with a number of patients and asked them how they would feel about answering questions and having a discussion about their own inhaler usage.

It is also important to appreciate the difference between professional learning and doing action research. Professional learning often takes the form of action learning; for example you could:

- initiate meetings for relatives and patients to get feedback from both parties and suggestions about how the service could be improved;
- set up brainstorming meetings among staff to solicit ideas about how to manage a ward better.

These would be action-oriented practice-based projects, but they would not be research projects because they do not fulfil research criteria such as gathering data and generating evidence. However, they can be extended to become practice-based research projects, as follows:

- Initiate meetings for relatives and patients to get feedback from both parties and suggestions about how the service could be improved. Keep records of activities and feedback, analyse the feedback to see if the initiative is contributing to better communication and producing concrete suggestions about how services can be improved.
- Set up brainstorming meetings among staff to solicit ideas about how to manage a ward better. Keep records of activities and feedback from the meetings, analyse and collate the data from the meetings, come up with new ideas and assess their effectiveness.

These days too many texts (even those that call themselves action research texts) stop at the level of action. This gives action research a bad name and also fails to promote the idea of nurses as educational researchers rather than only practitioners.

A key point here is that action research is educational in that people learn to develop a critical stance towards their own and others' learning. Critique is essential. Without critique we accept unquestioningly what we are told, and this leads easily into fundamentalism and stasis, themselves barriers to growth.

In summary, the main purpose of doing action research is to find ways to contribute to improving the social situation we are currently in. This calls for wise action, which begins with developing understandings of what we are doing within our particular situation and imagining ways in which it could be better. It means developing nursing knowledge, not only knowledge about nursing.

Now look at how you do action research.

How do you do action research?

Action research is a practical, common-sense way of understanding a practice thoroughly and improving it as necessary. This involves critiquing what is being said by others as well as what you have come to believe. You begin by asking, 'What is going on here?' This can apply to what is going on in the social situation you are part of, and also to your own thinking and understanding. For example, you may ask, 'Why have self-discharges increased over the last year in our unit?'

Action research is a disciplined, systematic process where you:

- review your current practice in the specific social situation you are in;
- identify an area you wish to study and improve;
- gather data about the existing situation;
- ask questions about how you can improve it;
- try it out and take stock of what happens;
- continue to monitor progress and begin to generate evidence;
- evaluate progress and establish procedures for making judgements about what is happening;
- test the validity of emerging knowledge claims;
- modify practice in light of the evaluation;
- explain the significance of what you are doing orally or in writing.

This process tends to take the general form of a cycle of action, reflection and modified action in light of the evaluation, as in Figure 1.1 (p. 15).

This notional plan can be turned into a set of reflective questions, as follows:

- What issue do I wish to investigate? What is my concern?
- Why do I want to investigate this area? Why is it important? Why am I concerned?
- How do I show the situation as it is? What kind of baseline data do I need to gather to do this?
- What can I do about the situation? What will I do? How will I do it?
- How will I gather data and generate evidence to show the situation as it develops?
- How do I check that any conclusions I come to are reasonably fair and justifiable? How do I test the validity of any provisional claims to knowledge?
- How do I modify my ideas and practices in light of my evaluation?
- How do I explain the significance of what I am doing? (see also McNiff, 2013; adapted from the original Barrett and Whitehead, 1985)

In practical terms, this means that you would:

- identify a particular concern or issue that you want to find out more about;
- gather initial baseline data to show what the current situation is like and show why the situation needs investigating;
- try out a different way of doing things;
- monitor what you and others are doing on an ongoing basis and continue to collect data;
- reflect on what is happening;
- generate evidence from the data and establish its authenticity;
- check out any new understandings with others;
- develop new practices in light of your findings that may or may not be more successful than previous ones;
- be prepared to explain to others the significance of what you are doing and its potential implications for others.

For example, you may wish to monitor and evaluate how well you are relating to patients and how they are responding to you, so that you can encourage them to believe in their chances of a full recovery. This is the basis of a person-centred approach to nursing (McCormack and McCance, 2010). Or you may wish to find ways of encouraging novice nurses to have greater faith in their own capacity for learning: this is the basis of an apprenticeship model of nursing. Benner (1984) outlines how nurses can develop from novice, to advanced beginner, to competent nurse, to proficient nurse, and finally to expert nurse. She makes the point that this is not simply about learning procedures but also about developing wisdom – a deep knowledge of what is involved in helping another person achieve a state of health that involves full engagement in life (see also Senge et al. (2005), who speak about the need for *presence* in practices).

A notional action plan could like this.

Identify a particular concern or issue that you want to find out more about

I need to check why Mr Brown is reluctant to start mobilising even though he had been walking unaided before admission and seems well enough to do so now.

Gather initial data to show what the original situation is like and show why it needs investigating

In my reflective diary I noted that when asked about this he was non-committal and said that he was rehabilitating well. One of my colleagues mentioned that he sometimes talked about his time in the army and showed quiet pride about his service. I noted this conversation too. When I was next changing his dressing I asked him about his experiences in the army and what he had learned. As he chatted it emerged that he felt it was unmanly to show weakness or dependency on others supporting him.

Try out a different way of doing things

During our next conversations I pointed out to Mr Brown the importance of developing strategies towards gradual independence and using the available support to ensure full independence. We agreed a walking frame would give him confidence to become more ambulant and that he could lessen its use as his confidence returned.

Monitor what you and others are doing on an ongoing basis: reflect on what is happening

Other staff and I observed whether Mr Brown was starting to walk short distances to the toilet and sitting room. We entered our observations on the nursing notes. I chatted with Mr Brown when I met him at various places around the ward and he seemed cheerful and confident.

Generate evidence from the data and establish its authenticity

The previous notes had referred to his lack of mobilisation. Now the notes constantly referred to his walking around the ward area. I selected those pieces of data that referred to his mobility or lack of it to show the situation as it developed and to generate evidence.

Check out new understandings with others

Colleagues and I agreed that we may have initially overlooked the value of simply listening to patients' own narratives and views. We felt that we could have used initial everyday chats with Mr Brown to learn more about him and his feelings about his present situation.

Develop new practices in light of your findings

We discussed at ward meetings the benefits of using everyday interactions in a more guided or focused way to help build up our overall picture of the individual person and their reactions to their present circumstances. This shows the importance of engaging dialogically with patients. It enables and encourages them to contribute to their own care plans and have a greater sense of agency.

The process of 'observe – reflect – act – evaluate – modify – move in new directions' is generally known as action-reflection, though no single term is used in the literature. Because the process is cyclical it tends to be referred to as an action-reflection cycle (Figure 1.1), and because it is open-ended, dynamic and transformational it may be known as educational. The process is ongoing because as soon as we reach a provisional point where we feel things are satisfactory, that point immediately raises new questions and it is time to begin again. In 1984, McNiff outlined her idea that action research processes can never be seen as straight, because issues may generate other issues, which may need to be dealt with before proceeding with the main issue. She produced the model illustrated in Figure 1.2 to communicate this generative and unpredictable aspect of action research.

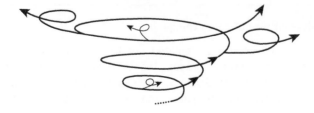

Figure 1.2 Visual to represent a generative transformational evolutionary system (McNiff, 1984)

Implications of these ideas are explored below.

3. WHAT ARE THE CORE ASSUMPTIONS OF ACTION RESEARCH?

Here are some of the most important assumptions of action research:

- Action research is values-based.
- Action research values and integrates all kinds of knowledge.
- This knowledge contributes to the generation of new theory.
- Action research is emergent and developmental.
- Action research is collaborative and inclusive.

Action research is values-based

Action research is values-based, and, like nursing, is always to do with care and respect for the other. This means it is democratic, egalitarian and ethical, because all people are valued equally. This idea is shown most strikingly in how people position themselves in relation to others, especially when explaining their choice of positioning as outsider or insider in the research. These ideas are developed in Chapter 3.

Action research values and integrates all kinds of knowledge

We said above that the aim of doing action research is to create knowledge and generate theory. However, it is important to appreciate that there are different kinds of knowledge; the main kinds are as follows:

- know-that;
- know-how;
- personal knowledge.

Know-that is also called propositional or factual knowledge and refers to knowledge about facts and figures. You test the validity of knowledge claims through pointing to empirical evidence: you can say, 'I know that today is Friday because it says so on today's newspaper'. Know-that is essential for nursing practices: you say, 'I know that patients need regular hydration', so you ensure that your patients get regular hydration. Knowledge of treatments and procedures is usually acquired from external sources such as books and other more knowledgeable people. It is also linked strongly with technical knowledge, which is essential for knowing about technology in patients' treatments.

Know-how is also called procedural knowledge and refers to skills and competencies and the application of procedures. It is a core element of nursing practice. Nurses need to build up their skills and expertise on a systematic basis. You demonstrate the validity of your claim that you are a skilled nurse by showing how you do things: you show that you can give an injection skilfully by doing it. Your evidence of the validity of your knowledge claim is in the testimony of your patient who says they didn't feel a thing.

Personal knowledge refers to the wisdom of practice and is linked strongly with common sense, built up through experience. It is also linked with the idea of your values: you listen to the inner voice that tells you what to do. Often nurses work on intuition: they know what is the right thing to do at the right time and the right kind of words to use in a particular situation. Polanyi (1958, 1983) speaks about personal knowledge as the basis of wise practice. No one can teach you personal knowledge; you have to learn it for yourself. It is linked strongly with the Aristotelian idea of phronesis, that is, wisdom in practice.

When you do action research as a nurse you draw on all these different kinds of knowledge. You develop and use:

- propositional knowledge for knowing about a patient's illness and treatment;
- procedural knowledge for knowing how to treat a patient; and
- personal knowledge for knowing what is the right thing to do at the right time in the patient's interests.

No one kind of knowledge is better than another, and they are all integrated within a nurse's practice. Unfortunately in today's university-based nursing education, know-that is given priority over all other kinds. Professionalism is reduced to what you know rather than how you know it or how you use your knowledge. It is a narrow, barren epistemology, with a focus on pieces of information, while not recognising that you need a different kind of interpretive capacity, usually acquired through experience, to bring all the pieces together as meaningful wholes.

Knowledge contributes to generating new theory

It is understood that knowledge can contribute to the generation of new theory. The word 'theory' means, broadly speaking, 'an explanation'. If you say, 'I have a theory about nutrition and recovery' you are saying, 'I know how nutrition and recovery work' and 'I can explain why they work in this way'. There is nothing mysterious about the idea of theory. We all have millions of theories about the way the world works, and we are constantly creating new ones. For example, you might find through experience that it is wise to start medication rounds earlier to allow for interruptions and avoid hurrying, which can lead to errors.

As with knowledge, there are different kinds of theory, including abstract theory and personal theory (there are other kinds, too, which we will not go into here).

Abstract theory (also called 'conceptual' or 'propositional' theory) is the kind of theory usually found in textbooks. As with propositional knowledge (know-that), it is the dominant form of theory used in universities. Nurses are expected to apply other people's abstract theories to their practices. These kinds of theories work from an idealised 'if only ...' perspective: Kant thought perpetual peace was possible if only people would behave in a certain way (see Bohman and Lutz-Bachmann, 1997). Habermas (1976) thought that an ideal speech situation would be possible if only ... and Rawls (1972) proposed a theory of justice that would work if only ... . These idealistic theories set out what a perfect world would look like. Unfortunately, they do not tell us how to get people to behave in such a way as to make the theory come true. To achieve this we need practical theories of real-life practice.

Personal practical theory is the kind of theory that people create for themselves. They study and monitor what they are doing, gather data to show the processes involved, and generate evidence from the data to ground their emergent claims to knowledge. You could say, 'I have come to understand why it is important to turn patients regularly' and you can compare this knowledge with the theories you read in the literature about the need to turn patients regularly to avoid pressure ulcers. However, while practical practice-generated theory helps us understand and explain how to improve practice, traditionalist academics are unlikely to accept it as valid theory. Back to the politics of knowledge.

Action research is emergent and developmental

When you do action research you ask questions and look for new understandings, not for final answers; this makes it distinctive from traditional social science research that focuses on getting to an end point where all answers will be revealed. In action research you begin from where you are, wherever this may be: you ask, 'What is happening in this place at this moment?' and you take stock so that you can work forward from there. This idea mirrors real life: we are always in the middle of something, and each ending is a new beginning. It is the same in nursing, which begins with the patient in the here and now. When you research your nursing practice in action you ask questions about intriguing or puzzling situations, so you can work out a better way of doing things. You always start from where your patient is, not from where you wish they were, although you would have a vision of where you hope they will be – in full health and full engagement with life. You do research into your actions to help you get to where you wish them and yourself to be.

Action research is pluralistic, collaborative and inclusive

Action research has always been linked with the idea of popular movements towards democracy and social justice. Accounts of its historical development appear in Greenwood and Levin (2007), Noffke (2009), McNiff (2013, 2014) and others. Most commentators agree that action research has been around since at least the 1930s, in different contexts committed to collaborative working (see for example, Stringer, 2007). They also agree that authors such as Freire (1970) and Dewey (1963) provided a theoretical basis for action research, though they were not identified as action researchers. The name 'action research' became popularised during the 1930s and 1940s, primarily through the work of Lewin (1946), who emphasised the need for the involvement of all in work situations. So it is commonly agreed that action research is pluralistic: everyone is acknowledged as of equal worth and equal status, and should be free to pursue the kind of life they wish to lead in negotiation with others. This carries considerable implications for nursing, because it means seeing everyone, including patients, as people in their own right. It means prioritising patients' interests above the organisation's: this has major implications for what counts as appropriate practices in nursing, and especially what counts as ethical behaviours (Chapter 3).

We now turn to the purposes and uses of action research.

4. PURPOSES AND USES OF ACTION RESEARCH

Action research is today used around the world in different ways. Two of the most important are:

- as a form of professional learning;
- as a form of social and political activism.

Action research as a form of professional learning

These days action research is widely seen as a powerful form of professional learning. It has been particularly well developed in education, specifically in relation to teaching and pedagogy (Carr and Kemmis, 1986; Elliott, 1991), and is now becoming established in nursing and related disciplines (Higgs and Titchen, 2001; Higgs et al., 2011). When people do action research they transform traditionalist models of teaching (the idea that in order to learn you have to be taught) into models of learning (everyone can learn for themselves). This has huge implications for traditional forms of nurse education, which tend to be based on a model of teaching: even in episodes of self-directed learning there is still the assumption that the student will go to the existing literatures. When people do action research they investigate their practices at first hand, including how they learn, individually and collectively. Collaborative learning and researching is a great way for individuals to explore their capacity for knowledge creation together.

These ideas were given especial importance through the development of the new scholarship, an approach developed by Boyer (1990), who spoke of the need for university teachers to develop different forms of pedagogy and integrate different forms of enquiry. He talked about the need for a scholarship of teaching, which involved:

- a scholarship of discovery, when you find out facts;
- a scholarship of integration, where you put the facts in perspective and make connections across disciplines;
- a scholarship of application, where you apply what you find to new areas;
- a scholarship of teaching, which begins with what the teacher knows and transforms and extends it. In this book we argue for a new scholarship of nursing.

These ideas were complemented in 1994 by Gibbons et al. who distinguished 'Mode 1' and 'Mode 2' forms of knowledge production. In Mode 1 forms, they said, knowledge is seen as disciplinary, static and hierarchically ordered, whereas Mode 2 forms are diverse, dynamic and 'socially accountable and reflexive' (p. 3). Mode 2 forms of knowledge production focus on solving problems and improving practices, are relevant to specific social situations and can be adapted to future similar contexts; we can learn from what we are doing and we can develop and adapt our learning. These ideas about Mode 1 and Mode 2 forms are similar to those described by Rolfe (1998) who refers to Popper's 'two worlds of knowledge'. Popper spoke about 'World 3 knowledge', which could be 'found in books, journals and other publicly accessible media' (Rolfe, 1998: viii), and World 2 knowledge, which is about what people know about themselves but is not in the public domain (World 1 knowledge is about knowledge of objects). Rolfe emphasises the importance for nurses of distinguishing between World 3 and World 2 kinds of knowledge:

Scientific World 3 knowledge tells us how patients with a certain illness *tend* to respond to a particular treatment, whereas personal World 2 knowledge allows us to look beyond the illness to the patient himself [sic]. (1998: viii; italics in original)

Professional education requires the integration of all forms of knowledge.

Action research as a form of social and political activism

This idea that all people can learn has special implications for nursing because it means that nurses and their patients and families may be included in debates about what counts as nursing knowledge and practice, and how these can be used for the benefit of all. This development is part of wider world movements towards increasing democracy and the inclusion of all people, including those on the fringes of mainstream society.

> In his Masters dissertation (2006), Odd Edvardsen tells the story of how he and his colleagues worked with local nurses and medics to set up a chain of survival networks in Kurdish North Iraq, to help them develop the skills and knowledge to support themselves. He writes:
>
> > My study shows the importance of having a network of actors who are deeply rooted in the local context in which one operates. In this way the intervention can develop according to the villagers' needs. This close contact with the realities of the villagers has made it possible for the project to develop according to changes in the injury panorama and also to start taking care of all those who have been exposed to injuries. The need to increase their competence has brought the chain of survival into the local health institutions. The challenges in the future will be to implement the model within the framework of the public trauma care system in the province. (Edvardsen, 2006: 3)

A major implication of the above is that action research and nursing are both real-world, living processes; they are always changing and have the potential to influence wider change processes. They are also always socially-oriented, and are therefore political because deliberate human interactions are always political in one way or another. This has considerable implications because it raises questions about how we understand processes of change, how we position ourselves in relation to other people, and how we understand the purposes of our work as nurses and researchers.

These aspects are explored further in Chapter 2, where we speak about why nurses should do action research, and whose interests this serves.

SUMMARY

This chapter has outlined what you need to know about action research. It has first considered what is involved in all kinds of research, followed by descriptions of how action research is distinctive, how you do it, and some of its core assumptions. Some of the purposes and aims of action research have also been identified.

The chapter has outlined ideas about knowledge claims, researcher positionality, the differences between professional development and action research, and the values-oriented nature of action research. The chapter also explains how action research can take the form of social and political activism.

Reflective questions

- Are you clear about what a knowledge claim is? Can you explain why critical reflection is important, and how this can enable you to articulate the significance of your research?
- Can you say what action research is and what it is not? Can you explain the differences between action research and professional development?
- Are you reasonably confident about how to do action research? What different methodological steps are involved? Can you comment on whether they are flexible or fixed?
- What are some of the core assumptions of action research? In what way are these different from the core assumptions of conventional social science research?
- What do you think are the purposes and uses of action research? Would you use action research? If so, when would you use it? Why would you use it?

TWO

Why should nurses do action research?

This chapter is about why clinical nurses should research their own practices as part of their everyday work. By doing so they can offer explanations for what they are doing and why they are doing it. They can show how their work is grounded in authenticated evidence, thereby demonstrating their capacity as researchers who are competent to make judgements about what counts as nursing knowledge. By doing action research and producing their accounts of practice, clinical nurses can develop a new knowledge base of nursing. A knowledge base comprises all the texts spoken or written about a subject; a new knowledge base of nursing would be grounded in real life accounts of practices, and so contribute to a reconceptualisation of nursing and nursing knowledge.

It is critically important to celebrate clinical nurses' knowledge and capacities. Nursing is a wonderful profession that aims to save lives, preserve dignity, provide comfort in illness, and ensure that people retain their humanity up to the point of death: this sets nursing apart from other health-related delivery professions (Cummings, 2012; Von Dietz and Orb, 2000). Most clinical nurses work hard with limited resources and often within restrictive bureaucratic systems whose focus is often on rationalising. However, the current situation in the UK and elsewhere is that nursing is under fire, as reported in Francis (2013). This has contributed to a widespread drop in public confidence in nursing and the low morale of nurses. Yet while recommendations are made about how to remedy the situation, few commentators identify the heart of the problem as rooted in the profound slippage between the espoused values base of nursing practices, which promotes patient-centred, compassionate care, and the current epistemological base of the nursing profession, which promotes technical rational ways of knowing and objectivised, one-dimensional practices that are divorced from feelings such as care. This in turn has led to a fragmented system where knowledge and practice are at odds with each other, with serious implications for the allocation of resources including labour and finance, and concerns for the quality of patient care. Nursing itself is in poor health, and for it to move back into its rightful wholeness, it needs to re-locate itself within a different epistemology, this time an epistemology of emergence and wholeness.

This chapter considers these points and is organised as follows:

1. Identifying the root of the problem.
2. Developing new practices and new thinking through action research.
3. Contributing to a new scholarship of teaching and learning for nursing.

1. IDENTIFYING THE ROOT OF THE PROBLEM

We argue throughout that the nature of the epistemological base of nursing could be seen as the root of the problem, and we develop our argument as follows.

Consider the relationship between values and practices. Values can be understood as transforming our principles into real-life practices: a commitment to freedom means that we try to honour the right of all people, including ourselves, to be free. Sometimes our values are denied in practice, and this can result in considerable dissonance. The point we now wish to make is that the underpinning technical rational values that inform what is accepted as nursing knowledge transform into and encourage technical rational forms of practice, and it is these forms of practice that are getting nursing into trouble.

To pursue this idea further, consider the terms 'epistemology', 'theory', and a new term, 'logic'.

Epistemology, theory and logic

We said in Chapter 1 that the term 'epistemology' refers to a theory of knowledge, a theory of knowledge acquisition or creation, and a theory of testing the validity of knowledge claims. We also said that there are different kinds of knowledge. The main kinds generally acknowledged in the literatures are technical rational (similar to 'scientific'), procedural (to do with skills) and personal (also called 'tacit' or 'intuitive'). All forms of knowledge may be seen as useful depending on the purposes of the people who wish to use the knowledge. Some people think it is possible to separate forms of knowledge from one another (which would give you a divisive form of epistemology). People who think like this would perhaps see reading reports of blood levels or ECG results as a technical rational activity, where you simply read off measurable and objective information. The reality is, however, that you need procedural knowledge to read and interpret results, and tacit and experiential knowledge to appreciate what this means for the patient.

In reality, all kinds of knowledge are integrated. However, in the dominant technical rational epistemology that underpins nursing, they are separated, because the kind of theory (considered next) that is most valued in mainstream nursing is conceptual and abstract, located in the head, not in the hand or in the practice. Forms of knowledge are also ranked hierarchically, where the epistemological system places technical rationality at the top, skills-based know-how at a lower rank, and intuitive forms at the bottom (Table 2.1).

Now to theory, and a reminder that the word 'theory' means, broadly speaking, 'explanation'. A theory of nursing explains what nursing is, how it is done and why it is done this way. The main form of theory promoted in the nursing literature is conceptual and abstract, located in the head. This means you can offer a theory of oxygen administration without actually administering oxygen, and you can theorise nursing practices without being a practising nurse. The form of theory tends to see things in a pure, idealised way, whereas real-life practices are far from pure and ideal. On the contrary, they are always contested and open to multiple interpretations. Shortly we begin to use the word 'agonistic', which is often used to describe difficult, problematic matters.

Add to the mix the idea of logic, which refers to how we think, which informs how we see the world. Some people use a linear, structured form of logic that sees everything moving towards a definitive answer. Other people see things as emergent and developmental. A misleading message in the culture is that there is only one form of logic – a technical rational form – that works in terms of outcomes and results, so this comes to be seen as the 'correct' way of thinking for all people. A reality check, however, shows that many people use an intuitive, relational form most of the time. Do you do what your GPS tells you or do you sometimes go on intuition? There is no one right way of doing or thinking, though the literatures try to persuade you that there is.

Different paradigms

These ideas about knowledge, theory and logic are usually described as constituting different paradigms. A paradigm refers to a set of ideas about knowledge, theory, logics and practices. Kuhn (1996) explained how paradigms shift and new ones emerge as part of historical and traditional processes. Currently, around the world, many cultures and disciplines are coming out of a deeply technical rational paradigm and moving into a relational paradigm. Some authors identify these new paradigms as postmodern (Rolfe, 1998); others such as Reason and Rowan (1981) simply talk about 'new paradigm research'. Action research is part of new paradigm research, because it is about real-world learning and thinking, instead of only analysing existing knowledge. We make the case in this book that the new paradigm research community needs to move towards a dialogical paradigm (see also McDonnell and McNiff (2013) on a new paradigm for sales and selling).

Sadly, official nursing knowledge is still stuck in old paradigm technical rational thinking, thereby limiting its options for development, with severe consequences for patients and nurses. It is still assumed that you can talk in abstract terms about nursing as a discipline without doing practical hands-on nursing. Dunne (1997: 25) says that such a view is futile: it is impossible to survey a social situation with impartiality because we are always already involved in the situation we are surveying. It is not possible to separate knowledge from knower. However, this continues to be the case with nursing. Discussions about what counts as 'proper' nursing and 'proper' forms of nurse education have moved away from where the patients are and into the universities. This has far-reaching implications for decisions about who counts as a nurse, what counts as nursing and nursing knowledge, and what counts as patient care (this theme is developed shortly). From a systemic perspective (including theoretical, practical and organisational perspectives), the entire contemporary system of mainstream nursing is organised hierarchically within and across domains, according to the dominant technical rational epistemology, with implications for objectivised and alienating ways of working, as shown in Table 2.1. This table is meant to show trends, rather than be taken as a literal representation.

Table 2.1 Hierarchies of knowledge across practice domains

	Form of knowledge	Form of theory	Role and status	Location of knowledge	Communication and acquisition	Uses of knowledge	Relationships
Most acceptable	Technical rational	Academic	Medics	Universities	Didactic	For the profession	Distanced, leader-oriented
Middle	Practical	Interpretive	Academic nurses	Hospitals	Autocratic	For the institution	Collaborative, team working
Least acceptable	Personal	Personal	Clinical nurses	At the bedside, in the home	Personal collaborative	For the patient	Personalised, dialogical with patients

The question now arises, how is it that nursing education has moved into the universities, and what are the implications for nursing as a practice? To appreciate how this has happened, look at this brief history of nursing.

Historical changes in the structures, focus and delivery of nurse education

Up to the 1970s, nurse training was conducted in hospital-based schools of nursing. Student nurses often lived on-site, were seen as part of the workforce, and spent much of their on- and off-duty time in the hospital milieu. There were disadvantages in this: service requirements could often come before training, and student nurses could be exploited. In the 1970s and 1980s nurse training was moved to separate colleges of nursing education, geographically set up away from practice settings. This separation between the physical locations of nurse training and the areas of practical activity signalled a break in the relationships between service and education. From this point, student nurses began to be seen as 'visitors to' or 'guests of' the hospitals, rather than an intrinsic part of the team.

About this time the 'Nursing Process' began to be introduced throughout hospitals in the UK. This was an attempt, designed in the US during the 1950s (Alligood and Tomey, 2010) to systematise the delivery of nursing care. It had many advantages as it moved from a task-orientated structure to one that emphasised the total care of a patient. It also clarified the responsibilities of each member of staff and identified the primary nurse for each patient. A disadvantage was that, as implemented, it required nurses to spend a good deal of time recording information about patients, which took them away from actual care delivery.

Around this time, during the 1980s, the separate colleges of nursing were subsumed into universities. Nurse tutors became university academics and the academic requirements for the recruitment of students were raised. The focus shifted more towards academic qualifications and away from the interpersonal capacities of nurses. As nurse educators moved into the university system the emphasis, having first been on service, then on training, now shifted towards the acquisition of abstract knowledge. An advantage was seen to be that student nurses were 'saved' from being exploited as part of the workforce. Unfortunately, this also lost numerous experiences that contributed to students' situated learning (Lave and Wenger, 1991).

Nursing care was carried out by three groups of nurses: (1) Registered Nurses, who took a three-year training course with a balance between practical and theoretical knowledge; (2) Enrolled Nurses, who took a two-year more practice-based training course; and (3) unqualified healthcare assistants, previously called nursing auxiliaries or nursing assistants, who had minimal training: 'nursing' has now been removed from the title. One of our research participants commented:

> During my time I have been called a nursing auxiliary, then a nursing assistant. I am now called a healthcare assistant so the word 'nursing' has been removed from my name badge. I sometimes feel this is a subtle way of pushing me further away from the professional centre of nursing. It struck me that many of the new nurses don't necessarily see care as central to their work. Maybe that's my corner of the market.

Further divorcing the profession of nursing from hands-on care, the role of Enrolled Nurse was dispensed with during the 1980s. Enrolled Nurses, whose training emphasised the development of practical experience were regarded by many as the backbone of the Health Service. Many had undertaken further training and education and become Registered Nurses, the highest form of qualification for nurses. Now, therefore, there was a large gap between the academically qualified Registered Nurses and the untrained healthcare assistants who carried out much routine care.

Also, during the early 1990s, the United Kingdom Central Council of Nursing and Midwifery (UKCC) introduced an altered scheme of training for registration; this new system was called Project 2000. Following academic selection, student nurses now spent most of their first year based in a university setting, engaging in academic study, more and more of which was self-directed. After this they would spend time in clinical areas as supernumeraries, usually working 9am–5pm for one or two days a week. This further separated the students from experiential learning and continuity of relationships with patients and relatives. Some students would reach the end of their first year's nursing education only to find that they could not tolerate exposure to the physical and emotional rudiments of nursing care, even as observers. Many traditionally trained nurses complained that this system turned out poorly qualified registered nurses who did not relate to the basic needs of patients. Over time, the system changed to one that allowed more clinical placements for the student nurses.

Currently, the overall pressures on the health service have increased the demands on nurses' time and made it more difficult to give a good standard in all aspects of care (Tovey and Adams, 2001). The continual policy changes within nursing, further activated by the nursing governing bodies would seem to have contributed to a situation where basic human care is delivered less readily than before. More and more this has been identified by horrific newspaper headlines, investigations and anecdotal evidence.

This has been recognized at UK government level, and one recent suggestion is that nurses should spend a year working as untrained healthcare assistants before entering nursing education (Triggle, 2013). This suggestion takes no account of limitations in employment budgets, and misses the point that if the system of education is not changed it is not clear who will provide information and leadership for the assistants. The ethos will remain unchanged and people will learn bad practices early. It also misses the point that knowledge has been increasingly systematised as technical rational forms, which means its validity may be judged in terms only of functionality and organisational use value.

So, what is the situation now regarding what counts as nursing and nursing knowledge, and the research base that produces this knowledge? Who counts as a knower, and who says so?

What counts as nursing?

The term 'nurse' is a protected title in the UK. To use it you must have an accepted nursing qualification. Entry to a course of study leading to this qualification requires certain academic qualifications. Therefore, given that much of the activity that the public would refer to as 'nursing' is carried out by healthcare assistants who have no such centrally recognised qualification, it follows that much work referred to as 'nursing' is actually carried out by people who may not use the term 'nurse'. Much of the care and direct hands-on help given to patients cannot therefore officially be called nursing. Defining nursing becomes increasingly problematic the farther up the technical rational ladder the profession of nursing climbs, consistently moving away from the direct hands-on care and assistance which nurses have traditionally prided themselves on doing so well.

What counts as nursing knowledge?

The kind of knowledge that is valued, now mainly in universities, is academic conceptual knowledge, generated by doing scientific and social scientific research. Much knowledge development work that could take place in day-to-day interactions in clinical environments is being missed because nurses and those studying for a nursing qualification are less involved in the work. Intuitive or experiential knowledge is generally regarded as unscientific and is therefore less valued. Instead of developing a language for understanding qualitative holistic aspects of care, the language used is only about measuring that which can be measured; further, if it cannot be assessed quantitatively, its existence should be ignored. Consequently huge amounts of research capability and knowledge development are allocated to a lower echelon in the order of thinking.

Who counts as a knower?

Only people who readily relate to the required orthodoxies of knowledge are therefore selected to become nurses. The strength of nursing moves into the quantitative scientific domain and out of the practice context. Such decisions are made unilaterally by senior-level bureaucrats: candidates are selected according to whether they can use an appropriate form of discourse, which by definition helps to decide the direction in which nursing moves.

Such practices render the system untenable, while the real needs of people continue and must be met at some point. It is, to cite Dyrberg (1997), a great example of the circular structure of power whereby a system perpetuates itself according to its own self-legitimation, excluding others and excluding critique. The consequences, however, are that such a system is non-sustainable and implodes, which is the situation in nursing today.

However, if this is the way things are, they can change. First, things don't have to be like this, though they will probably not change in the short term because it can be difficult to change entrenched systems. Second, attitudes and practices can change by introducing new thinking that may influence those systems.

The next section presents ideas about potential new options, and what can happen when clinical nurses adopt a critically reflective research perspective to their work and begin to contribute to new practices and new thinking.

2. DEVELOPING NEW PRACTICES AND NEW THINKING THROUGH ACTION RESEARCH

This section sets out why nurses in all contexts – clinical, organisational and academic – should do action research. The main purposes of action research are:

- to contribute to new practices: this is an action focus, where we try new ways of helping patients;
- to contribute to new nursing knowledge and theory: this is the research focus where we evaluate the effectiveness of changed practices and thinking;
- to contribute to a new scholarship of teaching and learning in nursing.

All aspects are intertwined and interdependent.

However, one of the main obstacles to developing innovative ways of thinking and practising is the mindset of many clinical nurses themselves. It seems to be the case that many nurses tend to feel comfortable with the idea of contributing to new practices, given that nursing is a hands-on practical profession, and accounts exist to show how people are developing innovative practices (for example, Jacobs, 2006; Meyer, 2006). However, like other practitioners, many practising nurses may not feel comfortable about being positioned as a theorist. Some are suspicious of the idea, having been researched on by official researchers. Many nurses we spoke with made comments such as the following:

> I have enough to do running my own clinical area, looking after patients, meeting targets and trying to keep everyone happy at the same time. I don't see it as my job to do theory. Isn't that what academics are paid for? We put it into practice when it comes to us though it doesn't always work in our area. Then we find later that someone has rewritten the book and contradicted themselves. Ah, well.

These perspectives are perhaps understandable, yet in practice they get the nursing profession nowhere. It is essential for practitioners to get involved in theory generation; nor is theory generation difficult since it involves offering explanations for what we are already doing. The public acknowledgement of nurses as practice innovators and theory creators is vital if clinical nurses are to be seen as legitimate participants in public debates about what counts as nursing and who counts as a nurse (Chapters 4–7 give advice about how to do this). However, public acknowledgement begins with the private acknowledgement of nurses themselves that they can contribute to new practices and new forms of theory. It is no good expecting other people to value your potential and your work if you do not value it yourself. You need to appreciate the importance of your work and your capacity to generate both new practice and new theory, as well as seeing how this has potential for influencing new directions in policy formation and implementation.

Two important points arise:

1. The importance of seeing yourself as a capable practitioner.
2. The importance of seeing yourself as a capable theorist.

The importance of seeing yourself as a capable practitioner

In Chapter 1 we set out Schön's ideas about the topologies of professional landscapes, which still, sadly, describe everyday practices in nursing. This can change by: (1) reconsidering what the work of practice-based nurses involves; and (2) considering how this might be achieved.

What does the work of nurses involve?

We said above that nursing is a wonderful profession that aims to save lives, preserve dignity, provide comfort in illness, and ensure that people retain their humanity up to the point of death. It is therefore important for nurses to be clear about how they think critically about what health means and what it involves. It is especially important that nurses are confident that they do not have to adopt a traditional medical model that sees patients from a deficit perspective, as outlined here.

Different models of health and health promotion exist in the literatures. The two main models, sometimes with variations, are:

- **A biomedical model:** the organism is understood as disabled because of disease or pathology of some kind, a view that stems from a traditionalist medical model. Underpinning assumptions are that there is an ideal state to which all are entitled, and it is the responsibility of health providers to help the patient achieve this ideal state. Health is defined in terms of absence of disease. Critics suggest that this model focuses only on changes in the individual's physical condition and ignores social contexts such as the interactions of the individual with society. To the credit of the medical community, many doctors, including General Practitioners, have abandoned this model in favour of more holistic perspectives, as outlined shortly.
- **A social model:** it is assumed that the individual is disadvantaged by social and/or environmental interactions and conditions. The broad assumption remains that 'full health' is the normal state of people. It is also assumed that it is society's responsibility to avoid circumstances that may further disadvantage potentially vulnerable people. Critiques are that the model ignores the fact that the individual themselves may be responsible for their own problems: perhaps they do not relate well to others and so further disadvantage themselves.

The work of nurses is therefore to provide some kind of 'intervention', help the person overcome their disabilities, and restore them to full health.

A critical perspective suggests that these are conceptual models of health: they exist in the head but not necessarily in real life. Things could be perfect 'if only ...'. But life is not like this. The philosopher Isaiah Berlin (1990) spoke about 'the crooked timber of humanity'. He said that people are not 'perfect', and it is a conceptual error to believe that we are or can be. It then becomes a practical error to try to turn people into 'perfect beings'. 'Perfection' is an idealised state imagined by people who like to think in idealised terms (the basis of conceptual theory). Instead, researchers such as Mouffe (2013) and Gray (1995) advocate a more agonistic perspective. It is futile, they say, to think that there is one kind of overarching universal law for everyone, given that, if we believe in pluralism, we have to accept that everyone is different. Perfection is impossible since it implies an 'ideal type' approach, so we just have to live with our imperfections and flaws.

This more realistic view informs a different model of health, termed 'salutogenesis' by Anton Antonovsky (1979), which maintains that people always live in contexts that are complex, unpredictable and somehow contested. He also uses an agonistic philosophy, beginning from the assumption that nothing is perfect. Even to think in terms of 'perfection' is to live in a fool's paradise, as well as being potentially dangerous, since it denies the very state of being human. Antonovsky's perspective maintains the importance of individuals developing a 'sense of coherence': they need to recognise what is happening to them, interrogate whether constraints are internal or external, and work, individually or in company with others, towards the most realistic and achievable state of wellbeing. From this perspective, the person is encouraged to exercise their agency in overcoming difficulties and move to as optimum a state of wellbeing and engagement as possible, what Czikszentmihalyi (1990) calls 'flow'.

While we do not subscribe wholly to the idea of 'salutogenesis', we do subscribe to its underlying philosophy regarding the physical, psychological and social complexities of human being and living and the need for as full an engagement as possible. This requires a recognition that 'normal' does not imply 'perfection', itself a dangerous and disabling perspective (and a product of conceptual theory) that suggests we all have to strive towards an impossible and unachievable state, and are therefore automatically doomed to failure.

Nursing practice is grounded in the idea of agonistics, including the contested nature of daily living, the problematics of what it means to be healthy, and the complex, unpredictable and frequently intuitive and unorthodox work of nurses. Nurses need to appreciate that they work in a constellation of practices, that they are part of the lifeworld of patients and have a duty of care to support them in achieving as optimum a state of wellbeing as possible. This involves working with patients from the perspective that we can all exercise our agency to the best of our ability to achieve the best possible sense of autonomy and coherence for all. It is not only patients, the traditional 'recipients' of care, who benefit, for in caring for others we care for ourselves. We are in this life together, and it is our collective responsibility to try to make it as egalitarian and productive as possible for all.

These views have consequences for how nurses relate to patients and to one another. One consequence is to advocate for a dialogical approach towards nursing. A senior nurse commented:

> By necessity student nurses are taught about how different disorders affect different people and the correct procedures to help them. In real life, with more experience they realise that few patients come in with only one condition, and the competing needs of those conditions are what complicates nursing care. A patient could have COPD (chronic obstructive pulmonary disease), diabetes and renal failure. The patient's own experience and personality are in practice the starting point for giving care. They know how they feel, they know what has worked for them before, and they can express the sort of preferences and biases that we all have in life. So it's important to listen to the patient and family rather than only interviewing them with a standard set of questions.

A dialogical approach towards nursing

As people sharing the world with other people, we should ensure our interactions are dialogical. This approach contributes to embedding education in the practice. Key theorists of dialogue include Bakhtin (1986), Bohm (1996), Buber (2002) and Macmurray (1957, 1961). A main principle is that dialogue is core to respectful, successful communication. According to Bakhtin (1986), all utterances happen in response to previous utterances, without necessarily aiming for closure. Each person in the encounter anticipates that the other will respond in a way that will keep the dialogue open. For Bohm (1996), this is the difference between dialogue and discussion. Discussion, he says, breaks things up: it 'emphasizes the idea of analysis, where there may be many points of view, and everybody is presenting a different one – analyzing and breaking up' (p. 7). He also contrasts dialogue and monologue, which adopts a different stance. In monologue it is not necessary to question one's fundamental assumptions (a requirement of dialogue). Often people who say they are engaged in dialogue in fact talk past each other. For Bohm, dialogue is:

> a *stream of meaning* flowing among and through us and between us ... out of which may emerge some new understanding. It's something new, which may not have been in the starting point at all. It's something creative. And this shared meaning is the 'glue' or 'cement' that holds people and societies together. (1996: 6, emphasis in the original)

Nor is dialogue simply about words. It means adopting an attitude of being prepared to listen to the other. This involves a particular frame of mind, anticipating that the other has something important to say, and being critical of one's own responses to them. Often, when we talk with others, we focus on what we wish they would say, rather than hear what they do say, and perhaps do not say. In a nursing context patients will often not say things; they will not tell you what they are thinking or what you need to know. It is then your responsibility to respond to the patient so that they feel confident that you are listening and taking them seriously, actively trying to understand. It means moving into the other's space and meeting them on their terms, not yours.

Now consider the importance of communicating these ideas to others, which positions you as a theorist.

The importance of seeing yourself as a capable theorist

When you suggest ways in which things could be different or better you are potentially contributing to new theory, because you are putting ideas into the public domain that possibly no one else has come up with before. Even if others have had the same ideas, individual outcomes will be different, and this acts as the basis of new theory. These are your ideas, your original contribution to knowledge of your field; other people can now learn from you and incorporate your ideas into their thinking if they wish. You contribute both to the practical world by offering ideas about new practices, and to the intellectual world by offering your explanations for those practices. Edward Said (1994) speaks about the importance of practitioners seeing themselves as public intellectuals. We are all intellectuals, because we can think for ourselves and communicate our innovative ideas. We can all do research and generate new theory.

Two strong implications emerge, about the right to research and the responsibility to research.

The right to research

Appadurai speaks about different public perceptions about who qualifies to do research:

Research is normally seen as a high-end, technical activity, available by training and class background to specialists in education, the sciences and related professional fields. It is rarely seen as a capacity with democratic potential, much less as belonging to the family of rights. In this paper, I will argue that it is worth regarding research as a right, albeit of a special kind. This argument requires us to recognise that research is a specialised name for a generalised capacity, the capacity to make disciplined inquiries into those things we need to know, but do not know yet. All human beings are, in this sense, researchers, since all human beings make decisions that require them to make systematic forays beyond their current knowledge horizons. (2006: 167)

Further, says Appadurai, all people have a right to research, 'to distinguish knowledge from rumor, fact from fiction, propaganda from news, and anecdote from trend' (p. 168). This, he says, enables us to find out what is important for others and ourselves. He speaks of the rights of every person to know what is going on around them and how they can contribute.

These ideas have special relevance for nurses, because what you know is special, and has special relevance for your patients and colleagues. You also have to keep up to date with the latest information and ideas about drugs and technologies as well as engage in ongoing learning about practices. You can learn these things only by researching the field, talking with others, reading professional literatures and being alert to new ideas.

This does, however, mean making a commitment to your own knowledge and capacity to create knowledge. Polanyi (1958) says that any act of knowing involves commitment to one's own capacity to know, while also accepting the possibility that one may be mistaken. Nevertheless, this should not prevent us from making our claims to knowledge with universal intent (Polanyi, 1958: 327), or saying that we have learned something with the intent of helping others to learn from our learning. This also involves ongoing critique to refine our learning as we evaluate it. Yesterday's knowledge about nursing practices is no good in light of today's knowledge innovations.

The responsibility to research

Nurses therefore have a responsibility to research, for several reasons. First, as noted, they have a responsibility to their patients and colleagues to stay up to date and ensure they are fulfilling their responsibilities to deliver high-quality care. Yet there is also a strong political reason why clinical nurses should do research.

Currently the majority of works in the public domain are created by academic university-based nurses. These works tend to speak about nursing at a conceptual level; they do not often engage with the everyday practicalities of nursing. This seems to be a regular phenomenon across the disciplines: elites identify themselves as spokespersons for the profession. Furthermore, professions tend to alter course to achieve new aspirations, which can move them away from the practical requirements of their client group, so some people's interests fall off the agenda. It is the syndrome challenged by Sojouner Truth in her 1951 question, 'Ain't I woman?' when she disputed the right of black women academics to speak on behalf of all black women. It is also the syndrome that nurses in clinical areas experience when they are spoken for and spoken about, especially, in this case, when their work, which focuses on patients, is misrepresented by a self-appointed ruling class whose focus is on academic specialisms. It is reminiscent of Marx's (1987) comment that 'They cannot represent themselves: they must be represented'. This is no good for anyone. Patients deserve to be treated by highly knowledgeable practical nurses who speak for themselves, and, where necessary, speak as advocates for their patients. The purpose of nursing must revolve around the needs of its client groups, the patients. It is the responsibility of the profession to deliver its expectations to meet those actual needs; it is not the responsibility of patients to move their needs closer to academic nurses' perceptions of what they wish to deliver. It is also vital that nurses do research in the interests of patients' and the public's perceptions and confidence. Currently perceptions of the role of a nurse are influenced by the same academic elites who own the nursing profession but who do not regard healthcare assistants, who actually do the routine work, as nurses. It is a case of occupational injustice, where workers are denied a sense of wellbeing through constructive participation in the workplace. Further, it is a case of representational injustice in that bright people are not allowed to speak for themselves.

Nurses need to speak for themselves. They need to exercise their political will to position themselves as professional knowers and engage with the politics of knowledge, knowledge production and knowledge dissemination. Producing accounts does not require writing in an artificial academic style, but clinical nurses do need to write for publication about their own experiences (see Chapter 8). Further, these texts need to be written with the authority of experience, and in a way that will be regarded as credible and scholarly. How you can do this is outlined in Chapter 7. Here we outline how this can make a massive contribution to the knowledge base of nursing practices.

3. CONTRIBUTING TO A NEW SCHOLARSHIP OF TEACHING AND LEARNING FOR NURSING

As outlined in Chapter 1, the idea of a new scholarship for teaching and learning began with the publication of Boyer's (1990) influential *Scholarship Reconsidered: Priorities for the Professoriate*. Initially it gained a firm foothold in the field of education, and has since gained widespread recognition within nursing, being adopted in 1999 by the American Association of the Colleges of Nursing (AACN), and achieving prominence on nursing degree courses in the UK and internationally. The key points emphasised in this New Scholarship are that 'scholarship' (or 'inquiry', or 'research') should be extended from its traditional narrow focus on academic scholarship to a broader focus that embraces practice and teaching. The idea has been taken up vigorously in many quarters and is widely seen as a democratisation of professional knowledge, in that practical knowledge is now recognised as of equal legitimacy as scientific and academic knowledge – at least, so the rhetoric goes, but not always the reality.

The democratisation of knowledge is a topic much discussed in further and higher education. Its interpretation in real life is something else, reminiscent of Chomsky's (1997) 'two models of democracy' view. Chomsky speaks about one model of participative democracy where people take an active part in negotiating and running their own affairs, and a second model of democracy (the current orthodoxy, which Chomsky calls 'spectator democracy') where people elect representatives to negotiate and run their affairs for them and then stand back and watch. This focus on spectator democracy, says Chomsky, is a symptom of a larger propaganda system through which ordinary people are persuaded to believe that they are not capable of thinking for themselves. The location of the New Scholarship in further and higher education could be yet another continuation of the same syndrome. The focus is still on 'the system', and the system is still organised hierarchically. Even though action research has entered official discourses, it is still largely a topic for scholarly debate. Practitioners' (especially clinical nurses') voices are seldom heard, possibly because of the public messages that practitioners cannot do research or generate theory and possibly because practitioners have come to believe those messages, and so refuse to engage for fear of being subjected to ridicule or other forms of silencing.

This can change, and must change. The professional knowledge of clinical nurses and healthcare assistants must be supported and legitimised; furthermore, they must be more proactive and take the opportunity to extend their own professionalism by developing their knowledge and expertise for their own benefit and for that of their patients. But to do this requires, as Schön (1995) says, that the new scholarship should develop a new epistemology. We suggest that this new epistemology needs to be dialogical.

A dialogical epistemology of nursing

In 1995 Schön made the point that the existing system of professional learning would never change unless institutions embraced what he called 'a new epistemology' – that is, a new way of knowing grounded in a new way of thinking (form of logic). This new way should be relational, that is, all people should be seen as in relation with one another, and with their environments. There is of course nothing new about these 'new' forms: they have existed throughout history, and are valid forms though they are not accepted as legitimate in mainstream higher education. At issue is how we make judgements about the validity and quality of practices. The mainstream criteria and standards used to make such judgements tend to be abstract rather than proceeding from a practical 'what works' perspective (Rorty, 2006). For example, formal guidelines for closing a head wound recommend the use of sutures; however, a strip of hair super-glued across the wound sometimes does the job just as well. In Cambodia workers in rural areas forged prosthetics for landmine amputees from spent shells and drainpipes (Vuthy et al., 2014), a practice that may be frowned upon in more formalised highly-equipped areas, but absolutely functional nevertheless.

What is 'new' in this new epistemology is an acknowledgement that the everyday practical knowledge of 'ordinary people' and workplace practitioners is as legitimate as formal propositional knowledge. This means therefore that 'ordinary people' and practitioners are as capable of knowing and creating knowledge as those who position themselves as 'official knowers'. However, given that practitioners have little hope of breaking into the strongly defended mainstream system, they need to develop new parallel strategies for getting their voices heard and promoting new criteria and standards for judging the quality of patient-centred practices and dialogical forms of thinking. Clinical nurses therefore need to develop an activist perspective to their work by developing expertise in communicating their knowledge, mainly through writing, in order to contribute to a new knowledge base for the profession, produced by nurses for nurses. Furthermore, they should be supported by academic practitioners who see themselves as practitioners who are working in higher education (see Chapter 9). This then avoids a 'them and us' scenario, but actively focuses on inclusional ways of being. It also includes patients and their families and carers to form communities of enquiry in the interests of all.

All this may seem rather grandiose and aspirational. It is not. Thousands of workplace practitioners across the profession have been awarded their masters and doctoral degrees for studying their own practices and producing their own accounts to show how they improved practices and contributed to a new knowledge base for their professions (for example, Binnie and Titchen, 1999; see also www.jeanmcniff.com/theses.asp). Nursing now also needs to get on board. This book offers advice about how this may be achieved, but, in the final analysis, it takes the political will of committed practice-based nurses to engage with the challenge and show what they can do.

These ideas are revisited in Chapters 8 and 9. But now a new wave of considerations enters the stage – that of nursing and research ethics. These matters are discussed in Chapter 3.

SUMMARY

This chapter has posed the question, 'Why should nurses do action research?'. It has discussed issues of epistemology, theory and logic, as well as the idea of shifting paradigms. A brief history of the historical changes in the structures, focus and delivery of nurse education has been outlined. The chapter also contains suggestions about why nurses should do action research from the perspective of perceiving oneself as a competent theorist as well as a competent practitioner. This would involve exercising the right to research, which brings with it responsibilities to research. By doing action research, nurses can contribute to a new scholarship of teaching and learning for nursing.

Reflective questions

- The chapter maintains that a technical rational form of knowledge is the basis of many of the problems in nursing today. Do you agree?
- Do you think that nursing is entering a new paradigm?
- Can you say why you should develop a view of yourself as a capable practitioner and a capable theorist? Why is it important to be both?
- Do you agree that all practitioners have a right and a responsibility to research?
- How can you contribute to a new scholarship of teaching and learning for nursing?

THREE

Ethical issues

Ethics is a core aspect of being an authentic practitioner-researcher, in nursing and in action research. In nursing you offer care and support to others; in action research you help people to think for themselves and develop spiritual connectivity. Ethics permeates all aspects of research, including choices about design and methodology, data gathering and interpretation, selection of participants, evaluation and dissemination of research findings.

Currently most nursing research adopts a medical model, conducted from within a scientific/social scientific outsider research paradigm, where some people are positioned as knowers and agents and others as recipients and subjects (see Chapter 1). In action research the situation is different because you work from a democratic and inclusional perspective, which requires an insider stance where subjective knowledge is valued. Outsider research can in fact be seen as profoundly unethical from an action research perspective, which regards all people as equal and as having the same inalienable rights.

This chapter outlines some core issues about ethics, including some of these kinds of problematics and critiques. It is organised as follows:

1. General information about ethics and ethical guidelines.
2. Some problematics and critiques.
3. Towards an ethics of action research for nursing.

1. GENERAL INFORMATION ABOUT ETHICS AND ETHICAL GUIDELINES

Nursing has its own official ethics guidelines, as does educational research (which is where many people locate action research). There is broad overlap between nursing and action research because both share the same philosophy and values base of care and compassion, and a desire for wholeness and full engagement with life (see also Hart and Bond, 1995: 4). Here are some of the official guidelines for nursing and educational research.

About official guidelines

Ethics is about what people believe is good. It refers to a system of moral principles about how people should live their lives in relation with others. In professional practices it also deals with matters of rights and responsibilities, what counts as right and wrong and good and bad, and how these matters are decided.

Conventional guidelines exist in codified form across disciplines and professions, including for nursing and action research. Most are legalistic in nature, based on the Universal Declaration of Human Rights and the Nuremberg and Helsinki Agreements, and emphasise the need for dignity and rights for all.

Ethical guidelines for nursing

The main code of practice and professional conduct for nurses in the UK appears in *The Code: Professional Standards of Practice and Behaviour for Nurses and Midwives* (Nursing and Midwifery Council, 2015). Professional responsibilities are identified as follows:

- The people in your care must be able to trust you with their health and wellbeing.
- Make the care of people your first concern, treating them as individuals and respecting their dignity.
- Work with others to protect and promote the health and wellbeing of those in your care, their families and carers, and the wider community.
- Provide a high standard of practice and care at all times.
- Be open and honest, act with integrity and uphold the reputation of your profession.
- Have appropriate arrangements in place for patients to seek compensation if they have suffered harm. (Nursing and Midwifery Council, 2014)

Bellman summarises the above as:

> The emphasis within research ethics is: the prevention of harm; maintaining confidentiality; ensuring informed consent; honesty and integrity; and the right to withdraw from the research project (or treatment). (2012: 147)

These guidelines have been supplemented by the so-called '6 Cs': care, compassion, competence, communication, courage and commitment. Nurses are required to internalise and implement these in everyday practices.

The situation regarding the importance of guidelines is different in nursing and research. In nursing, most nurses would act in the spirit of the guidelines in accordance with their own values base. In some circumstances, they may need to seek advice from senior colleagues about correct procedures, and appropriate advice would then be given according to established professional standards. In research it is different: your research would have to be vetted and approved by ethics committees, who police guidelines rigorously. This is when things begin to get tricky, because critiques show inconsistencies and contradictions within the guidelines themselves as well as raising questions about the ethical basis of different research methodologies (and the situation changes again in relation to action research, as outlined shortly).

Now we consider some official guidelines for educational research.

Ethical guidelines for educational research

Research guidelines are found in statements from national and other major educational research bodies. In Britain the main body is the British Educational Research Association (BERA) whose Guidelines state that:

All educational research should be conducted within an ethic of respect for:

- the person;
- knowledge;
- democratic values;
- the quality of educational research;
- academic freedom.

The main responsibilities of educational researchers are:

- Responsibilities to participants:

  o voluntary informed consent;
  o openness and disclosure;
  o right to withdraw;
  o children, vulnerable young people and vulnerable adults;
  o incentives;
  o detriment arising from participation in research;
  o privacy;
  o disclosure.

- Responsibilities to sponsors of research:

  o methods;
  o publication.

- Responsibilities to the community of educational researchers:
    - misconduct;
    - authorship.
- Responsibilities to educational professionals, policy makers and the general public. (British Educational Research Association, 2011)

Some action researchers have attempted to draw up a code of ethics for action research but none appears so far to have pursued this line of thinking seriously. Zeni (2001) says she abandoned efforts to do so, preferring to raise questions. We agree. We also suggest that clinical nurses themselves, linking with their practical research, should develop a personal and collective ethic of nursing practices, grounded in a practical evidence base, which they could make public through a new body of knowledge (Chapter 9). Demonstrating ethical conduct is not simply a tick-box exercise or the application of guidelines to everyday practices. It is far more complex, because we are talking about real-life people who all hold different values and try to live them in practice in their own way. It is said that simply to expect people to follow guidelines would be 'an imposition of a *status quo* by an institution' (McNamee, 2002: 8).

Further, we need to recognise that we are always situated in real-life, power-constituted complex contexts, so life is full of dilemmas, some of which cannot be resolved. This means we have to make choices about how to act. The idea of ethics and ethical behaviour therefore takes on real-life meaning only in the day-to-day realities of trying to live harmoniously with others. Further, the ethical choices we make extend to the methodologies we choose and how we position ourselves in relation to others. What we choose decides whether the entire conduct of the research and its design are ethical. Ethical conduct has to come from the heart, not from a list; it is a lived experience, not a paper exercise. Everyone has to work things out for themselves in negotiation with others who are doing the same, and explain what they are doing so they can show how they hold themselves accountable for their practices. This is where slippage happens between the theory of the abstract guidelines and the realities of everyday practices, and powerful critiques are launched, as we now discuss.

2. SOME PROBLEMATICS AND CRITIQUES

Here are three areas of problematics and critiques, in increasing levels of importance. Not surprisingly, the more important they are, the subtler they become. They are:

1. Internal contradictions within the guidelines.
2. The uncritical commitment to the application of theory to practice.
3. Different ethical standards regarding relationships in research.

Internal contradictions within the guidelines

Many of the guidelines are contradictory to one another. These contradictions can be understood more easily by considering two strong theoretical frameworks from Habermas, about (1) system and lifeworld and (2) knowledge-constituted interests.

System and lifeworld

In various texts, such as *Legitimation Crisis* (1975), Habermas speaks about 'system' and 'lifeworld'. The 'system' operates through rules and regulations, and is generally associated with institutions and other social structures. We often say, 'Blame the system' or 'I cannot change the system'. Within institutional systems people occupy roles and carry out job descriptions: many see this as sufficient to qualify as ethical behaviour. (NB: Habermas points out that systems are created by humans, which means that they can be recreated; but this brings conditions and implications, including the exercise of determined human agency, as we explore shortly.)

The lifeworld, on the other hand, is to do with practices and human interactions. It is always discursive, that is, it manifests throughout all our discourses, whether spoken or enacted. According to Foucault (1980b), any form of discourse or human interaction is potentially power-constituted. As soon as two people meet, some kind of power relationship is always waiting to emerge, whether emancipatory power or coercive power. Which kind emerges depends on the quality of the relationship and the intent of the people in the encounter. For Habermas, system and lifeworld are always in a mutual dialectical relationship, each informing the other.

This framework of system and lifeworld has implications for the interpretation of ethical guidelines. Consider, for example, the idea of 'do no harm'. Harm to someone is often unavoidable throughout life; you cannot please everyone all the time. Nurses often find themselves in conflict with the opposing needs of patients and relatives, and of the organisation and the profession. Consider, for example, the requirement for hospital staff to achieve targets for waiting times. Because of frequently extreme pressures, patients are sometimes left on trolleys in corridors before being admitted onto a ward to avoid their being recorded as statistics. At the time of writing the Accident and Emergency departments of many UK hospitals are in crisis because beds intended for incoming patients are already in use by patients who are well enough to go home, yet who cannot be guaranteed appropriate follow-up care in the community. Similarly, the required recording of achievement of targets can be misleading: sometimes a practice is not recorded if it does not confirm an anticipated outcome. In cases like these, the organisational bureaucratic managerialist system works against the practical lifeworld-oriented work of nurses. This situation is likely to persist if politicians continue to dismantle the National Health Service, leading to a fragmentation of services and a lack of joined-up provision of care.

Now consider the idea of knowledge-constituted interests.

Knowledge-constituted human interests

Knowledge, says Habermas (1972), is always related to human interests, and can be analysed as three separate but interlinked forms: technical, practical and emancipatory.

Technical interests

This refers to a researcher's desire to discover empirical facts about the world through the production of technical rational knowledge. The usual methodology is scientific investigation. In nursing you would aim to find out about a certain technique, for example focusing on the merits of a particular form of wound dressing. Technical rational knowledge is acquired through study of the objective world, mainly in order to understand, control and use it. Contemporary nursing focuses increasingly on technical rational forms of knowledge, often with a reliance on technology, which requires nurses to develop their understanding of the use of technology, sometimes at the expense of patients.

Practical interests

Practical interests focus on meaning-making and interpretation, with the intention of understanding the social lifeworld and developing critical awareness of its historical and political emergence. In nursing, this kind of knowledge is essential for interpreting events and experiences, and for developing sensitivity to people and contexts. This means more than, for example, the use of an appropriate form of language or awareness of individual differences; it is a state of mind that enables us to understand the relationships among people.

Technical and practical interests also often overlook matters of cultural sensitivity. We live in pluralistic, multicultural societies that are always culturally and historically situated: each group has its own complex and frequently conflicted history. Cultural sensitivity is frequently an issue for guidelines regarding consent and autonomy. Hammersley and Traianou (2012) comment that most adults are regarded as able to give consent, while children are not, and raise the question of 'children and adults who have disabilities that could affect their capacity to be informed or to consent in a manner that takes account of their own interests' (p. 10). They also comment on cultural differences that require different interpretations of the concept of autonomy:

> However, in some non-Western cultures ... the head of a kin group or a community leader may be regarded as having the proper authority to agree to whether members of the family or community should participate. Such cultural differences are important, and can pose difficulties: should the researcher respect the established culture or insist that individuals are fully informed and freely consent? Would that be possible? (Hammersley and Traianou, 2012: 10)

Similarly, when negotiating access to practitioners in workplaces, it is often assumed that getting permission from the manager is sufficient: the manager speaks for all (McNamee, 2002). While securing permission may have achieved formal criteria, and been approved by an ethics committee, the research itself would have been fundamentally unethical.

Technical and practical interests not only often overlook matters of cultural sensitivity and other forms of situatedness, they also fail to appreciate that the people who make judgements are themselves situated. For example, the authorities in the Victoria Climbié case failed to take action to save her from further abuse by her guardians who believed her to be possessed by demons. Social workers and police 'were reluctant to intervene, in part, because they did not know how to respond to the cultural complexities of the situation' (Midgley, 2008: 8; see also the Secretary of State for Health & Secretary of State for the Home Department, 2003). Many examples like this exist in the literatures, giving further reason to not take guidelines at face value or interpret them too literally.

Emancipatory interests

Emancipatory interests enable people to understand the influences that lead them to act and think as they do, and to liberate their own thinking to resist closure of any kind. In nursing it is essential to spend time thinking about the historical and cultural experiences of your patient so that you act appropriately. For example, in some cultural contexts it would be inappropriate for nurses to care for members of the opposite sex, while in others you should take care to leave an appropriate distance between yourself and another in a social situation.

Carr and Kemmis (1986) say that the aim of action research is to enable people to take transformative action, that is, to change the social situations they are in. This is all very well and to be encouraged, but exercising your right to think for yourself can be problematic. Instances of whistleblowing are regularly reported in the nursing literatures, when staff report organisational injustices or misuse of resources; reprisals are often so severe that nurses' careers are ruined. In February 2015, a new Francis Report, *Freedom to Speak Up*, recommends that whistleblowers are given appropriate support and protection and that honest and fair dealing should be encouraged organisationally. It remains to be seen whether these recommendations will be carried through, or whether the situation will remain as described by Alford (2001; one of the best texts from the whistleblowers literature), who reports former whistleblowers' advice as: 'Do it to save lives, otherwise don't do it. The costs are too high.'

Now consider a second set of problematics.

The uncritical commitment to the application of theory to practice

There is widespread criticism of the assumption that a direct relationship exists between recommendations and their implementation: that once something is in the head or on paper, it will be done. The assumption ignores the fact that those who are to implement the recommendations (in this case, practising nurses) usually work in intensely busy life-and-death practice contexts, where complex issues are not easily resolved, and often cannot be resolved. The guidelines remain what they say they are: they guide towards a goal. They are noble and aspirational in nature, what Hume (1985) called 'oughts' rather than 'is's'. Although most people would do their best to achieve them, this is not always possible in the world of human interactions with its contradictory demands and frequently irreconcilable differences.

Further, in this case, the abstracted form of ethical guidelines itself becomes unethical. It becomes what Lyotard (1984) calls a 'grand narrative', that is, a totalising narrative that accepts unquestioningly the stories that are put about in society and that end up governing our lives, including, for example, the stories that patients cannot think for themselves or that nurses cannot do research. These stories are often ideological in nature and are created by those in power with the intention of maintaining their power; a further example of Dyrberg's (1997) views about the circular nature of power. Lyotard suggests that the grand narratives that govern societies should be replaced with or at least be balanced out by local narratives, where 'ordinary' people working in real-life situations speak for themselves from their own situatedness. The issue of deciding whether what they say should be taken seriously may be negotiated through what Habermas (1976) calls 'intersubjective communication', that is, the making public and sharing of stories to see if they are appropriate for the specific culturally and historically constituted nature of the time and place. This sharing itself needs to be done by those who also share the same culture and history – that is, they are insiders and have what Zeni (2001) calls 'indigenous knowledge': they know from experience and from tradition what they are speaking about.

Now for a third assumption, at the heart of the matter.

The ethics of researcher positionality in different forms of research

Several texts are available that deal with issues regarding the relationships automatically assumed within different research traditions (for example, Campbell and Groundwater-Smith, 2007; Herr and Anderson, 2005; McNiff, 2014; Zeni, 2001). All explain how action research signals a break away from what Eikeland (2011) calls 'the othering business', that is, where conventional social science researchers position participants as 'others' in the research. He says:

> Certain ethical aspects, obligations and consequences are inherently implied in the basic structures and relationships of the techniques of both action research and mainstream social research, which are implicitly chosen by choosing one approach and not the other. ... One important such aspect concerns the question of who is included in the community of inquiry and interpretation, and what/who are the subjects of study. (Eikeland, 2011: 39)

He goes on to explain the importance of differentiating between communities of practice and communities of inquiry, and transforming the one into the other. Communities of practice, he says, contain people from all sectors and levels: indeed, the situated learning and communities of practice literatures (including Lave and Wenger, 1991 and Wenger, 1998) explain how communities of practice may be structured in terms of organisational and professional hierarchies, where managers and employees, and experts and novices, stay at different structural levels, albeit engaged in the same enterprise. Good examples from a nursing perspective are Benner et al. (1996, 2010) who recommend a situated apprenticeship model for nurses' professional learning (see also Sennett (2008) for compelling ideas about the need for apprenticeships in professional learning).

Communities of practice tend to work from a systems perspective, where the interests of the organisation are prioritised over those of the individual. Communities of enquiry, however, do not have these structural hierarchies because all become participants who are enquiring into their own practices:

> ... instead of a segregated 'we' ('them') of researchers studying 'them' ('us'), an expanded 'we' start to study ourselves: What are *we* doing to ourselves and to each other, how and why? (Eikeland, 2011: 39, emphasis in original)

This matter is central also to nursing practices and nursing research. In nursing practices, how do 'we' as nurses position patients, families and colleagues? In nursing research, which methodology do 'we' nurses choose to achieve the kind of person-centred values and practices that are currently being recommended in policy literatures (as in the 2012 Report 'Caring for Our Future': online at www.gov.uk/government/publications/caring-for-our-future-reforming-care-and-support)? We argue here that it is not enough simply to pay lip service to issues of ethics in practice and research, but also to have the courage to make critical choices about which research approach to use. This is especially important in action research, because it means being prepared for some of the inevitable personal, social and organisational fallout this will engender, and being prepared, intellectually and professionally, to deal with it. Here are some suggestions about how to do this.

3. TOWARDS AN ETHICS OF ACTION RESEARCH FOR NURSING

All practices are values based, none more so perhaps than nursing, which is always conducted in the immediacy of what it takes to be alive and well. People's lives and the quality of those lives are at stake. Authors such as Cuthbert and Quallington (2008) and Cranmer and Nhemachena (2013) are right to emphasise the importance of values and ethics in care practices, and authors such as Ghaye and Lillyman (2010) are right to emphasise the centrality of reflection in practice. Reflection means thinking about what you are doing. Arendt (1958) identified this capacity as the core of what it means to be human. She says that if we do not reflect on what we are doing, we become thoughtless, literally without thought. Alford (2001) says that the ability to talk to ourselves, and explain to ourselves what we are doing is an important part of our individuality. Without it our lives become meaningless and 'value-less'.

The idea of values refers to those things we hold dear, what we value. One of the dilemmas for nurses and professionals in general is to decide on their own values base, and which values to live by. A further and more difficult task is to justify those choices. The difficulty is demonstrated by comparing Gandhi and Al Capone. What makes one a saint and the other a sinner in popular perceptions? Both had strong values about social order, strong family values and strong ideas about emancipation (whose order, whose family and whose emancipation was another matter). How do we make judgements about why we choose certain values and not others?

Something similar is happening in the shifting values base of contemporary nursing practices. Perhaps even up to twenty years ago there would have been common agreement that the core value of nursing was care for the patient. Things have changed. These days, the word 'care' is actually disappearing from professional discourses, often to be replaced by terms such as 'skills' and 'capacities'. The caring base of nursing is being systematically erased from the profession. Given, as noted in Chapter 2, that the practical hands-on care of patients is provided by healthcare assistants, who are now becoming designated, even in public discourses, as 'carers' rather than 'nurses', questions arise about what counts as the values base of nursing and who sets its standards. Above all, responses to the question 'Who is nursing for?' remains contested.

The perspective we take in this book remains that nursing is about caring for the patient. This is not simply our words spoken in response to ventriloquist policy makers, but is born of a lifetime working in nursing and associated professions, and from the experience of doing action research within those professional contexts. But working with action research now presents new challenges, because if we are saying that nurses need to make their own decisions and test the validity of those decisions against the critical feedback of others, then nurses also need to set their own criteria for what counts as professional practices, and how they are to be judged. From an action research perspective, values transform into criteria for judging the quality of practices. But claiming the validity of the values base of practices, and claiming the right to do so involves at least two aspects:

- asking critical questions of self and others;
- negotiating with ethics committees.

Asking critical questions of self and others

Nurses need to ask themselves, and others, critical questions, including the following.

What values inspire your work?

When doing action research, it is important to be clear about the values you hold that inspire your work, and that you hope will transform into living practices. When realised in practice, these values become a form of applied ethics. Ask yourself the following questions:

- Why are you a nurse? What makes you do the job you do?
- What values inspire your work?
- How do you justify these values and not others?
- Are you prepared to compromise any of these values? If yes, which ones? If not, why not?
- Are you living your values in your practice? If so, how do you show this? If not, what do you do about it?

Engaging with questions like these enables you to explain how you are evaluating your work (doing evaluation means you do action research). You are testing the validity of your work, and also testing the validity of your judgements. Testing the validity of this capacity to make judgements enables you to claim that you are engaging in ethical practices: ethics means always questioning the rightness of what we are doing, holding the process of making judgements open to public scrutiny, and being prepared to change in light of more developed understanding.

What motives inspire your research?

Whose needs are you meeting in doing your research – your own, your patients', your organisation's? Sometimes people do research to meet institutional and personal achievement targets or to gain academic rewards. This is fine, provided the reasons are clarified from the start. Be clear about your motives and how you intend to carry out the research. Always check: is your research genuinely going to contribute to improvements for patients? Will you be publicly accountable? Will you involve all client groups such as patient bodies, health delivery organisations and professional bodies?

Which methodology do you choose, and why?

Aim to be clear about the underpinning assumptions of the methodology you choose. This means being clear about how you position yourself in relation to others, both in nursing practices and in research practices. Values inform your practices and your research; they transform into practices, and also transform into how we judge the quality of those practices. In action research we are always in equal and respectful relationships with others. Winter and Munn-Giddings comment:

> The guiding impulse of action research is the 'improvement' of situations involving a practical responsibility for others' wellbeing. So, immediately, its ethical basis is different from, and in some respects simpler than, the ethical basis for conventional research, where an ethical basis needs to be provided for 'purely experimental' activities which contrast sharply with responsibility for practical care. (2001: 220)

As Eikeland notes, action research has to be participative, otherwise it denies its own nature:

> … action research, as practised, is often simultaneously pulled in opposite directions, both towards standards set by externally based, academic research, and towards internal indigenous standards, creating ethical dilemmas. But action research can hardly let go of the indigenous standards without losing its soul and … [becoming] mainstream research. (2011: 40)

The same could be said of nursing.

But maintaining this focus on the participatory, egalitarian nature of action research (and nursing) requires nurse action researchers to check how they position themselves in relation to others in general. This poses a new question.

How do you position yourself as a nurse practitioner-researcher in relation to others, and how do you position them in relation to you?

As a nurse, and as a researcher, how do you see other people, and how do you position yourself in relation to them? Common typologies in the nursing literatures suggest that nurses might see the patient as a disease, a case or a person

(Liaschenko, 1997). These themes are well developed also in philosophy. Buber (1937) speaks about how you can adopt different positionings in relation to others. He speaks about an 'I–It' relationship, where we see others as an 'It', an object in our space, and an 'I–Thou' relationship, where we see the other as a person in their own right. This is not an 'either-or' situation: Buber explains how most of us move constantly between 'I–It' and 'I–Thou' stances. Bohm (1996) develops similar themes, and Macmurray speaks especially about the self as agent (1957).

These ideas have considerable significance for nurses. How do you position your patient, their families and yourself? How do you understand your own capacity for agency? Do your patients have agency too? Do you see them as the recipient of a procedure, someone who depends on you and others for their wellbeing, or as a fully engaged person, albeit currently disadvantaged because of their physical or mental circumstances, and who you can help get back to full engagement? How do you position yourself – as someone who has the answers to their problems and can do things for them, or as a collaborative colleague who can help them find ways of doing things for themselves?

The following story is told by two nurses involved in voluntary overseas work.

> We worked in sub-Saharan Africa. Our job as nurses was to train local individuals to provide some basic levels of care and advice. There were no doctors or hospitals for miles around. Our approach was conversational and hopefully respectful of local cultures. We always tried to put across that we wanted people to use their own local knowledge and experience combined with our nursing knowledge, so that it made sense in the environment. A problem we came across was that some individuals wanted to buy in to the western idea of medicine and set themselves up as mini-doctors and then tell other people what to do. Whereas we hadn't wanted to introduce any kind of hierarchy, some people immediately wanted to have power to themselves and we had to fight against this. They wanted to use their knowledge mainly to set themselves up above others and would imply almost magical powers for some of the everyday medications we could provide. It was frustrating for us who were trying to be egalitarian as we saw it but not everyone wanted to work that way.

How do you understand the nature of nursing knowledge?

How do you understand the different kinds of knowledge that inform nursing practices? Do you buy into the dominant epistemological system that values primarily (sometimes only) technical rationality? This approach tends to see people as separate entities. The aim of practices is to achieve final solutions, which involves developing skills and competencies. In this book we maintain that all kinds of knowledge are appropriate for nursing practices and inform different epistemological stances. While skills are an essential aspect of nursing practices, they need to be balanced with other capacities, including empathy and wisdom in knowing which skills to deploy at any specific time. This means moving from techne to phronesis, from technical rationality to wisdom in practices. Phronesis is rooted in an inclusional epistemology that sees all things as constellations of interrelationships, all in a process of emergence towards new forms.

How do you judge the significance of your nursing practices and your research practices?

A core philosophical idea is that of beginnings rather than endings, of continuous learning rather than arriving at final answers. A key author here is Arendt, who speaks about the idea of 'natality', which refers to the idea that, through their birth, each person brings something new to the world. The idea is extended through appreciating how, every time we take action we also set in motion a series of beginnings. The fact that we take action is a statement of intent to shape the future. A salutogenic model of health (Chapter 2) and an action research methodology are premised on the idea of beginnings. Nurses and patients, working and learning collaboratively, ask, 'How do we manage this current situation in order to bring a better future into being?'.

Asking questions like these have significant implications for the attitudes and practices of nurses.

However …

Negotiating with ethics committees

However, it is all very well to claim the right to identify values as criteria by which we judge the quality of practices, but what about when we appear before conventional institutional ethics committees and review boards? These bodies continue to work according to the conventional research guidelines outlined above. How to negotiate your personal guidelines and official guidelines?

This calls for political strategies, so here is some advice. The points are extended in Chapter 7, so they are noted here only briefly.

First, aim to show the quality of your research. You can do this by demonstrating awareness of methodological matters as well as suggesting new procedural ones.

Methodological matters

These include:

> **The research shows internal validity:** Does the proposal or research you present to an ethics committee demonstrate authenticity? Does it show how

you are living your values in your practice? Does it show your engagement with appropriate literatures? If it does, you can claim that the research demonstrates internal validity.

The research shows methodological rigour: Does the research show that you have observed methodological steps, from identifying a research issue to claiming that you have engaged appropriately with the issue? Does it contain quantitative as well as qualitative data as appropriate for the situation, and correct procedures for data analysis? Does it show how you have tested the validity of your claims against the critical feedback of knowledgeable others? If it does, it demonstrates methodological validity.

The research shows its use value for social good: Does the research show that it will have use value for individuals and for wider society? Can other people learn from it? Can they extend this learning to others, so that your research may be shown to have 'impact'?

The research makes an original contribution to knowledge of the field: Can you show that doing your research has enabled you to contribute new thinking and practices to knowledge of the field?

You can also negotiate procedural matters with the ethics committee. You could ask them, for example, to be prepared to do some prior reading about action research, or include some key papers with your proposal or research report. Most academics these days are aware that action research is here to stay, and many would be sympathetic to its philosophies, even if they don't do action research themselves.

Make sure also that you are fully prepared for ethics review meetings. Because you are still walking in new territory you need to be more prepared than normal, and possibly anticipate questions and challenges. However, don't anticipate trouble or create difficulties where they don't exist. People can often be more open to new ideas than expected.

SUMMARY

This chapter has outlined issues regarding ethical guidelines in nursing and in educational research. Some questions are raised regarding the value of guidelines like these, as well as some contradictions internal to the guidelines. Two important conceptual frameworks are offered: system and lifeworld and knowledge-constituted interests. A further important concept of researcher positionality is discussed. The chapter proposes an ethics of action research for nursing.

Reflective questions

- Are you familiar with general ethical guidelines for nursing and for research? Do you think guidelines are important? If so, why?
- As well as the problematic areas identified in the chapter in relation to ethical guidelines, please identify at least two more.
- Why are the concepts of system and lifeworld important?
- How do you understand the idea of researcher positionality? Why is it important?
- Is it possible to imagine an ethics of action research for nursing? Is it desirable?

II

HOW DO YOU DO ACTION RESEARCH?

This part explains how to do action research in a nursing context. It gives practical advice about planning and designing an action research project, including matters of feasibility in busy clinical settings. It outlines how to monitor practices, gather, analyse and interpret data from which to generate evidence to ground knowledge claims. This is important for demonstrating the methodological rigour of your research, and for claiming validity and legitimacy for your knowledge claims (dealt with in Part 3).

The part contains Chapters 4, 5, 6 and 7.

CHAPTER 4   PLANNING AND DESIGNING ACTION RESEARCH

This chapter outlines ideas about planning and designing action research. It identifies two broad areas of interest. The first is about doing action research in an organisational context, and considers strategic, process and feasibility matters. The second is about considering what it takes to become a researcher. Advice is offered regarding personal, practical and professional considerations.

CHAPTER 5   DRAWING UP AND CARRYING OUT ACTION PLANS

This chapter outlines how to draw up and carry out action plans. It gives advice about different approaches and models and how these might be realised in practice. Practical advice is given for different steps in an action enquiry, at different levels of progress. An example of an action plan is provided. A framework for drawing up a timetable or schedule for conducting an action enquiry is offered.

CHAPTER 6 MONITORING PRACTICES AND GATHERING DATA

This chapter deals with matters of monitoring practices and gathering data about them. The practices in question are identified as your learning, your actions, other people's learning and other people's actions. All are in transformational mutually reciprocal relationships of influence. You are advised to look for data in all contexts, and advice is offered about where to look for the data and how to gather them. Further advice is offered about how to manage the data, with alerts about some potential ethical and practical implications.

CHAPTER 7 TURNING THE DATA INTO EVIDENCE: TESTING THE VALIDITY OF CLAIMS TO KNOWLEDGE

This chapter outlines how to turn data into evidence. It revisits the idea of making claims to knowledge, generating evidence from the data, and testing the validity of the evidence and the claims. Ideas regarding matters of criteria and standards of judgement are offered, as well as information on how to analyse and interpret data for generating evidence. Advice is given regarding procedures for testing the validity of knowledge claims, and for validation procedures.

In the next part we go on to discuss the significance of your action research and its importance for suggesting new directions for the profession.

FOUR

Planning and designing action research

Before you begin your action research project or draw up specific action plans, ask yourself these questions:

- What do I want to research?
- Why do I want to research it? What is the point of the research?
- Who will benefit?

Also think about what you hope to learn that you don't already know, and what you will do with this knowledge. It is important to satisfy yourself on all these points so that you can approach others with confidence, especially in a nursing context, which is always busy, dynamic and person-intensive. Also remember that any provisional decisions you make about planning and designing your research need to be negotiated with others, both to gain their support and to ensure it is organisationally feasible.

Checking feasibility is key because you need to be clear: (1) whether you will be able to carry out your plans from logistical and organisational perspectives; and (2) whether you have the capacity to do the research in terms of motivation, stamina, access to resources and negotiating a work–life balance.

This chapter addresses these issues and is organised as two sections:

1. Doing action research in an organisational context.
2. What does it take to become a researcher?

As noted earlier, nurses are expected to do research, perhaps for continuing professional development requirements or for degree or ongoing accreditation. However, how 'research' is construed depends on the political context of the organisation you are working in:

- If you are in a traditionalist context, 'research' may mean simply being 'research aware' or 'research literate' (see Chapter 2). It may also mean being involved in research from a conventional research stance, where you become data in another researcher's project, or gather data for them.
- If you are in a more progressive context you will be actively encouraged to do research with an expectation that you will contribute to organisational learning or even to policy formation and implementation. This can be exciting though demanding. Much research in clinical settings is part of educational programmes and is frequently self-interested. Research gets more support from everyone if benefits can be seen for a wider group of people.

Also remember, should you decide to do an action research project, not to stop at the level of doing something that looks only like problem solving. Make sure you do research. This means remembering the difference between action learning, where you learn from, say, trying out a new idea or strategy, and action research, where you study what you do, generate evidence through gathering and analysing data and articulate the significance of the experience. This is where action research also goes beyond professional development, which emphasises actions but not always the reasons and purposes for the action. Action research is about showing that claims to improved practices must be interrogated and justified. It is about praxis, which is informed, committed action that gives rise to knowledge as well as successful action. It is informed because you take other people's views and feelings into consideration; it is intentional because you examine and interrogate the values that give rise to the research, and you are prepared to defend them. Praxis also demonstrates wisdom, phronesis, in Aristotelian terms, and not only techne, which is to do with technical rational knowledge and a focus on outcomes.

1. DOING ACTION RESEARCH IN AN ORGANISATIONAL CONTEXT

Doing action research in an organisational context means understanding organisational dynamics and developing interpersonal and negotiation skills. Especially it calls for understanding the relationship between the individual and the organisation, and how to negotiate a balance between organisational and personal interests and values.

Thinking about organisations

All organisations are made up of individuals, and working as an organised group of individuals can mean different things to different people. Organisations tend to work in terms of roles and responsibilities, which are usually arranged as structures. Some of these structures work in terms of hierarchies and some as dynamic democratic networks. In many cases the organisation becomes seen as a free-standing entity with its own values and interests, and takes on an identity of its own, which may or may not reflect the values base of its members.

Organisations have their own cultures. Most organisational development literatures emphasise the value of collaborative and cooperative working. They also speak about the use of power in organisations, whether from the top when it often becomes authoritarian power administered by those in charge, or through collaborative working patterns when it becomes the organisation of positive forces negotiated by all members of the organisation. The action research literatures show how practitioners can exercise their power and influence for personal and organisational change.

The relevance for you is that a well-designed action research study can and often does bring benefits to all: patients, nurses and caring staff, the organisation and the wider profession of nursing. By developing new knowledge and new practices from which others can learn, your research can have a ripple effect, bringing maximum benefit to others. Therefore it is important that you learn how to manage yourself so that you can develop your capacity for research and exercise your educational influence in other people's learning.

Planning and designing an action research project means thinking about:

- strategic issues;
- process issues.

Strategic issues

Strategic issues tend to focus on the following (you may come up with other areas specific to your context):

- Identify and articulate the research area and the research issue.
- Identify and articulate research goals.
- Offer a rationale for the research.
- Identify potential stakeholders and participants.
- Imagine strategies for demonstrating and ensuring wider impact.

Identify and articulate the research area and the research issue

Be as clear as possible about which area and which issue you hope to investigate. This might be inter-professional or inter-disciplinary communication; organisation of the day involving decisions about how many nurses will be available for morning or afternoon shifts; or the direct contribution of hands-on care to patients. Coghlan and Brannick suggest:

> Before making a final decision [about which issue or issues you will investigate] you are well advised to reflect on each issue identified from personal and organizational perspectives with a view to establishing:
>
> - the degree to which it offers an opportunity to experiment with existing and/or newly acquired knowledge;
>
> - the degree to which it offers opportunities for personal growth and learning;
>
> - the degree to which issue resolution offers the possibility of increasing your profile within the organization;
>
> - the balance between personal gain and organizational gain in the event of successful resolution;
>
> - the degree to which the issue may be resolved within known resource and time constraints. (2001: 83)

A strong benefit of action research is that you look at the situation you are in and the people you are with, and observe how benefits radiate out immediately to others rather than have a trickle-down effect. Hart and Bond (1995) say that a benefit for nurses doing action research is the 'change agent' role they adopt, where they are able to create alliances and open up spaces for others also to become change agents. Whatever area you identify, be as clear as possible about what you wish to achieve and in whose interests you are doing it, whether for yourself, your colleagues, the organisation, or the patient. For example, from an organisational perspective it is important to achieve quicker discharge times for patients, because it improves the organisational figures and standing, though it may not necessarily be in the patient's interests. Or you can seek to make professional claims to knowledge of direct benefit to the profession, such as an improvement in nursing strategies that can lead to an enhanced patient experience. However, while benefits for the organisation and the profession are important, it is more important to see the patient as the centre of gravity. Everything done in an organisation needs to be done in the interests of the patient.

Identify and articulate research goals

Identify and articulate your research goals, and the reasons and purposes of your research. If you are doing a higher degree course this would include ideas about making original contributions to knowledge of the field and the generation of new theory. Aim to articulate a clearly defined research question. In action research this often takes the form, 'How do I understand and improve my work?' In traditional social science research it tends to be reasonably straightforward to show whether research goals have been achieved by looking at anticipated outcomes and results in terms of other people's changed behaviours. In action research the outcomes often take the form of personal learning and practice improvement.

Offer a rationale for the research

Research is always undertaken with intent, to do with creating knowledge and generating theory for the benefit of others. In nursing this means primarily for your patient and their families. Research is always political. You ask, 'What do I need to know? Why do I need to know it? What will I use my knowledge for? How will I explain the significance of my knowledge?' (see below). In action research, where action and research come together, you aim to improve the quality of your action by investigating it and coming to understand it more deeply, so that the action itself improves through research. You learn how to provide better patient care through studying how you provide patient care, and find ways to improve what you are doing.

Identify potential stakeholders and participants

Action research is always collaborative, which has implications for you. You need to liaise and negotiate with others, including your line manager, about how you can work within existing organisational structures. Remember that your organisational manager may not be a nurse (they are possibly a former supermarket manager), so is removed from the professional line of reporting. It is therefore especially important to make a case for the research in organisational terms. You may need to negotiate between organisational interests and your professional nursing interests. This is something people in organisations have to do on a regular basis. Nurses are subject to multiple pressures from different directions, which can make life difficult (see Figure 4.1).

Generally, the principle stands that if a patient will benefit from your research this should also satisfy any organisational or professional questions. Aim, therefore, to identify possible benefits to the organisation, the profession and to patient care. Also identify possible negatives, problematic areas and likely difficulties, such as possible staffing implications, need for additional time to do the research (your own and perhaps other people's), and possible resource implications. You will need ethical approval for virtually every area, and especially if you wish to involve patients in your research. This raises issues about which kind of data you hope to gather, where you will get it, whether you will be granted permission to get it, and which criteria you will identify for analysing and sorting the data to generate authentic evidence.

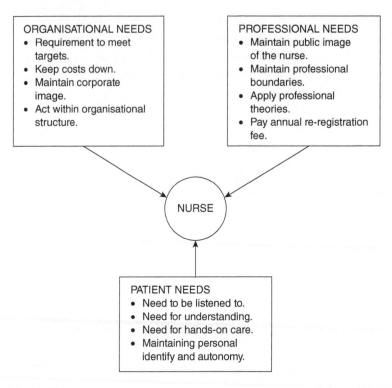

Figure 4.1 Multiple pressures on nurses

The issue of involving patients can be problematic, although this has central priority for improving the quality of nursing, as recommended in The King's Fund report *Patient-Centred Leadership: Rediscovering Our Purpose* (The Kings Fund, 2013). Check whether you can involve patients and relatives and get their feedback, and be prepared to allow sufficient time for negotiating this. The experiences of some researchers indicate that the time taken can vary widely (Ah-See et al., 1998). Many of the problems in nursing arise because we don't ask patients. Stay aware, too, of the need to make judgements about potential negative effects, by, say, exposing the vulnerabilities of patients. Consider, for example, whether there is already a high anxiety rate, or whether the patient's intellectual performance has been affected by procedures. Informed and equal consent must be addressed in terms of the patient being fully informed while bearing in mind the power differential between patient and nurse, even if this exists only in the patient's mind. Remember that if you solicit a response from a patient they will probably be anxious to please you by giving what they think would be the 'right' answers. Also make sure that the people you are working with know that they should be informed about the research and can withdraw permission at any time. Bearing all these cautions in mind can be problematic. Bellman (2012), citing Streubert Speziale and Carpenter (2007), comments: 'The action researcher should anticipate as many of these tensions as possible, although it may not be possible to identify them all'.

When negotiating working relationships remember that you are trying to achieve shared aims, which means also respecting the professional boundaries of medical and other staff. Take into account duty rosters and the fact that life goes on when you are not there. You need the full cooperation of nurses and other colleagues. As with all activities, research is more successful if carried out in a climate of positive participation.

Imagine strategies for demonstrating and ensuring wider impact

A major issue these days is the idea of demonstrating research 'impact', though it is not always clear what this means. Some people create definitions to suit their own purposes. It is relatively easy to do research that produces findings that suit a small group of people, or that support the views of professional leaders or reinforce existing orthodoxies. These findings do not always offer a complete picture of the situation and its contexts. 'Impact' is a slippery concept. Nevertheless, you do have to imagine some way by which you can make judgements about practices and performance, and there are many perspectives from which this may be done. Nurses can judge their own performance and other people's performance by identifying criteria that help to test the validity of knowledge claims, and people from other disciplines can give feedback (see Chapter 7). Patients can also gather data and offer feedback, and thereby become co-researchers. This is important methodologically, in that triangulation is a central aspect of gathering data, to show perspectives from multiple points of view (see Chapter 7). The wider the angle of enquiry the more authentic the research.

To achieve this, build in regular feedback mechanisms to stay on track. Report to your key collaborators including fellow nurses, senior professionals and non-nurses in the professional and organisational line-management system. Remember that the research will probably develop in unforeseen ways, so it is impossible to have a specific plan for rolling out. However, to keep sight of your aims, stay flexible and remember that you know more today than you did yesterday and that this new knowledge can change situations.

Now think about process matters.

Process issues

The process issues considered here are:

- participatory planning;
- addressing the priorities of stakeholders and participants;

- negotiating institutional support;
- managing your time.

Participatory planning

This section sets out the main principles of working with others, and identifies the main groups of people you would probably work with and the kinds of discourses needed for successful collaborative working.

Groups of people

In Chapter 3 we emphasised the importance of being aware of how you position yourself in relation with others and any potential influence on your working relationships and patterns. Whether you really do include others as participants, as 'we' or one of 'us', also decides the ethicality of your research. This means you would aim to include your colleagues, line manager, patients, relatives and carers as research participants. If you are on a higher degree course you will also work with your course tutor and other course members, some of who may act as critical friends or validation groups. When planning your project check its feasibility with them to ensure they will support you, and check their availability to know when you can call on them. Participants are vital resources for the success of your project, so aim to treat them well. Take stock of how well you manage your interpersonal relationships. If any area needs improving, work at it until participants' responses tell you that you are succeeding. In particular, aim to develop interpersonal skills, including the capacity for listening carefully and responding appropriately. Learn to listen to yourself as you speak with others and check especially whether you are using an inclusional form of language.

Addressing the priorities of stakeholders

One of the benefits of doing action research is that it is directly relevant to real-life problems and issues. You do not have to dream up a research topic: you are in the project situation at every moment. As soon as you ask, 'How do I sort this out?' or 'How do we develop better ways of working?' you have begun to research your practice.

Identifying and prioritising research participants' issues is important because the practice of nursing is always done on behalf of other people. You judge the quality of your practice in terms of how well you contribute to your patient's autonomy and independence of mind wherever possible. Say you work with an athletic person who is in hospital for a serious leg wound that needs regular changes of dressing, and is about to be discharged. You could experiment with the patient how to dress the wound such that they had reasonably full mobility and could change the dressing themselves. At all times attend to the needs of the patient.

Negotiating institutional support

If you are working in an institutional setting such as a hospital or nursing home it is essential to gain the support of others including your managers, colleagues, patients and their families. This means asking yourself critical questions about whether they will lend support, and how you can manage your relationships so that it will be given. If you are working independently you also need to ensure you gain the support of any colleagues such as co-team nurses, your patient and their families or carers. Questions about the feasibility of your project would include:

- Will everyone support your efforts? Aim to keep everyone informed about your research plans and progress, so that you do not appear simply to be doing your own thing, or spending too much time writing up your journal when you should be helping with the workload.
- Check all issues raised earlier – opportunities, negotiating constraints and conflicts of interest, access and permissions. Also check allocation of time and resources.
- Make sure you always conduct yourself professionally and with courtesy. Respect conventions and stay on top of everything.
- Respect the cultural climate. Be sensitive to whether people are open to new ideas or are possibly defensive. Aim to be enthusiastic without being pushy.
- Be on good terms with your manager. Try to find out how your manager thinks about research and deliberately set up conversations with them.
- Be aware of how you are positioned within your institution and in relation to others. What is your functional role? Will your research help or hinder you and others? How can you communicate to others your enthusiasm for research, and your desire to develop an institutional research culture?
- Negotiate access to resources. Check whether you have access to, say, photocopying facilities, use of institutional computers and resource centres, support from librarians and technical assistants. Check whether you can negotiate additional time for your research; this would probably depend on whether your institution is committed to supporting a professional learning culture, and especially whether clinical nurses are supported in doing research.

Managing your time

Check also whether you may have access to additional study time. Time management can often be an issue: doing research always involves additional time – reading, maintaining a diary, gathering and sorting data, talking with participants, or drawing up ethics forms. Sometimes organisations encourage nurses to do action research and make time for it during the working day, but sometimes individuals or groups may become hostile or resentful of the time taken during the normal working day. A manager has been known to say, 'If you have time to write, I can find you some work to do'.

Deciding to do your research takes careful consideration. What can you negotiate with family, friends and colleagues? What is negotiable in your life, and what is non-negotiable? Make sure you get your work–life balance right. Prioritise family time and make time for relaxation. Take a walk through the park. Whatever you decide, just be aware that you are going to have to dip into personal time, and do not complain later.

We have considered some of the things involved in working in an organisational context. Now think about what it takes to be a researcher and how to develop your own research capacity. These matters are especially important if you are on a continuing professional development or an award-bearing course.

2. WHAT DOES IT TAKE TO BECOME A RESEARCHER?

Doing research can be exciting and also demanding. Planning and designing a research programme requires you to think about who you are and what you stand for. Many things are involved in becoming a researcher, but here are some main considerations, at the personal, practical and professional level.

Personal considerations

Be prepared to do the following.

Change your identity and mindset

Becoming a researcher means seeing yourself as able to do research and generate theory. This can be difficult for many nurses who automatically think of research as written in capital letters, something other people do. This kind of thinking moves research away from the practice setting and puts it into the hands of only academics and scientists. It can be difficult to change self-perceptions, especially when you come to believe the rhetoric that says nurses cannot do research. However, it

but needs other people for its meaning to be assessed' (Fry, 2014: 32). These ideas are important for nurses who enable patients to use their knowledge to speak and act for themselves, or to advocate for them if they are unable to do so. Elliott comments:

> In 'action' conditions are created that enable the agent and others to reveal their individuality and uniqueness by starting something new and, in doing so, to transcend what is merely required of them in their roles in life. If 'action' has an aim, it is to enlarge the space in which human beings can relate to each other as unique individuals in the situation. Such an aim is not the intention to produce an outcome or result, but a value built into the process of action itself. (2003: 9)

- How will I check that it is useful knowledge? Useful for whom?

Doing research means testing the validity of knowledge claims by identifying specific criteria and generating evidence from the data that show the criteria in action. This acts as the basis of judgements about the usefulness of research and its knowledge outputs. In nursing the quality of the knowledge is assessed in terms of its benefits to the patient. These matters are developed in Chapter 7.

Through engaging with these kinds of questions you are able to make a valuable contribution to knowledge of your field, which is nursing practices.

Practical considerations

At a practical level, be prepared to do the following.

Read widely

If you are on a course you are expected to read widely and engage with appropriate literatures. When you read you meet authors who are speaking about their ideas. This gives you the opportunity to test your own ideas against theirs. Through engaging with their ideas you are able to develop new ideas and evaluate your own perceptions. You can also identify important theoretical frameworks for your study such as patient autonomy and occupational justice. These concepts become armatures and structures around which you can build arguments and new constructs. Reading also helps you to engage with your own thinking. You get to know what you are thinking through adopting a reflective stance where you distance yourself from your thinking and critique it.

Reading the ideas of others also helps you to check any conclusions you come to against the evidence in the literatures and offer reasons for a range of issues, including your choice of methodological approach, positioning as outsider or insider, strategies for ensuring ethical conduct, choice of criteria, and many other issues.

Aim to factor your reading into your study time. Aim to read something serious for an hour each day, even if this is in five-minute slots. Read on the bus or when standing in a queue. Electronic devices can be invaluable: download texts from the Internet to read in odd moments.

Access information from any available source. Use the library if available; use the Internet and social networking, hospital archives and public reports. Read critically and challenge normative assumptions, including your own.

Work closely with your supervisor

If you are on an award-bearing course you will be assigned a supervisor. You may also be assigned a professional tutor in your workplace. Aim to work with them, not against them. Always do assignments on time and professionally. Do not turn in work that is less than perfect – this means producing an error-free, technically and conceptually accurate text. Aim to meet your supervisor regularly and keep all appointments. Supervisors are on your side and expect high standards from you. Treat them with respect; they are officially allocated a very small amount of time for supervision purposes, and most spend far more time and effort than they should, so be fair with them and develop a mutually respectful professional relationship.

Maintain good records and produce regular progress reports

Aim to maintain good research records to keep yourself and others informed. This means keeping a research diary or journal, and a reflective journal, which will become part of your evidence archive. These are confidential to you but be prepared to make them available for official scrutiny if and when necessary, especially when you attend supervision sessions or periodic assessments. Aim to maintain records regularly and keep them up to date. Playing catch-up is difficult, so maintain discipline and procedure to ensure that data is updated continuously and regularly. This also helps to ensure accuracy of recording and avoid unnecessary reliance on memory. Keeping others informed enables them to make judgements about the quality of your work, make suggestions and give feedback or raise critical or problematic issues in real time. Aim to maintain goodwill, and keep everything above board, so that professional conduct is seen to be carried out.

Also aim to produce regular progress reports and make these available to your professional tutor and academic supervisor. Good record keeping and report writing are important from professional practice perspectives and from research perspectives; this is how you keep records of your research practices, reflections and learning.

Draw up action plans and time lines

There are many different ways of approaching an action enquiry, and different books offer a range of advice. We have found that the best action plan is where you ask yourself questions about what you wish to do. These act as a set of prompts to keep you on track. Chapter 5 offers extensive advice about this.

Professional considerations

At a professional level, aim to do the following.

Develop an appropriate language

When you are in a clinical setting you speak a clinical language. You speak about diagnoses and care plans. When you are in a scholarly setting you speak a scholarly language. You speak about epistemology and theory. Scholarly language should be clear and accessible as well as scholarly and formal, that is, it needs to show the characteristics of scholarly activity. These include issues of analysis and interpretation, critical engagement and testing the validity of findings. It is important to develop the right language for the right context. Achieving the cognitive switch from clinical language to scholarly language takes practice and time. It also involves a conceptual switch, where you re-identify yourself as a scholar as well as a practising nurse.

Engage in scholarly debates

Developing an appropriate language and mindset enables you also to engage in scholarly debates. This is essential when you write essays and dissertations for academic accreditation. When you produce a text it has to show that you have engaged at the level of ideas, not only at the level of clinical practice, and that you are able to theorise what you are doing, not only describe it. Theorising means analysing practices and suggesting why and for whom they are significant. It enables you to claim that you are a competent theorist as well as a competent practitioner.

Be prepared to write

Being a researcher means writing reports, papers and dissertations. Over time it also means writing for journal publication and producing books. Writing does not often come easily to people, even to the most experienced writers. Contrary to popular opinion, good quality writing takes a small amount of talent and a large amount of hard work. This means working at your craft and developing expertise, which takes time, commitment and patience.

That said, writing is one of the most important things you can do to promote ideas about the need for patient-centred nursing. When you write you move through different spaces at increasingly significant levels of influence. You transfer what is in the head, in a cognitive space, onto the page, in a rhetorical space, and into the world, in a political space (Sharples, 1999). You use writing to develop yourself as an intellectual activist where you are able to show the practical activism involved in working with and for patients, and offer strong theory-based, evidence-based reasons for doing so. You can also articulate the significance of what you are doing for patients' wellbeing and for the future of the nursing profession. These ideas are explored further in Chapters 8 and 9.

SUMMARY

This chapter has outlined ideas about planning and designing action research. It has identified two broad areas of interest. The first is about doing action research in an organisational context, and considers strategic, process and feasibility matters. The second is about considering what it takes to become a researcher. Advice is offered regarding personal, practical and professional considerations.

Reflective questions

- Have you a good sense of what is involved in planning and designing action research? What are the main issues?
- What do you need to watch out for when planning to do action research in an organisational context?
- What are the main issues in becoming a researcher? What do you need to think about?
- What feasibility matters do you need to think of when designing action research? Will you be able to carry out and complete a project? What circumstances might help or hinder you?

FIVE

Drawing up and carrying out action plans

Now that you have thought about practical, methodological and ethical issues, you need to draw up an action plan with a view to taking action and researching the processes involved. This chapter offers advice on how to do this, highlights some dilemmas to watch out for and maps the advice onto a real-life story to show the process in action.

The chapter is organised as four parts:

1. Drawing up your action plan.
2. Practical advice for carrying out your action plan.
3. An example of the action plan in action.
4. Drawing up a schedule for an action enquiry.

1. DRAWING UP YOUR ACTION PLAN

An action plan acts as a guide to engaging with the question, 'How do I improve my practice?' (Whitehead, 1989). You explain why this is an important question, and why you should engage with it. Your action plan is flexible, in the same way as a road map is flexible: alternative routes are suggested, anticipating that unexpected events may arise, so be prepared to adapt and change course as appropriate. Your action plan acts more as a series of prompts to keep you on track and maintain sight of your end goal, which in your case means an improvement of practice and the capacity to explain in what way it has improved and what makes you feel justified in saying this. Also remember that the word 'improve' does not imply that something is bad. It means that you evaluate your work at every step of the way. If it needs changing in some way, you take steps to improve it. If it is already as good as it can be, you explain why you think this is the case and offer justification for your reasons. Unless you focus on improving things all the time, you will in fact stand still because life will run ahead of you. Your practice will never be 'best'; even Olympic champions practise all the time. What you hope for is that your practice will be as good as possible for this particular moment in this particular context.

The question, 'How do I improve my practice?' or 'How do I improve what I am doing?' often arises from a situation where your values are denied in your practice. If you work in practice development in nursing, for example, you may like to think that you are facilitating work groups in a democratic and supportive way, but then find on reading participants' feedback that you are suppressing their feedback through a rather authoritarian stance. As a community nurse you may wish to arrange occupational therapy services for a patient but then find that the service is not available in your district. How do you resolve the dilemmas? What do you do?

Here are some ways in which you can imagine developing a course of action. First, look at this set of ideas from Barrett and Whitehead (1985):

• I experience a concern when some of my values are denied in my practice.
• I imagine a solution to the problem.
• I act in the direction of the imagined solution.
• I evaluate the outcome of the solution.
• I modify my practice, plans and ideas in light of the evaluation.

The same ideas appeared, in different words, in the work of Dewey (e.g. 1963). Dewey was an American pragmatist philosopher who believed strongly in the need for the authentic participation of all in social and political life. He believed that living is a form of enquiry where you constantly investigate interesting and important dilemmas, a view that has led to the contemporary concept of problem-based learning and that has informed the work of major theorists such as Kolb and Kohlberg. Also note that 'problem' for Dewey did not mean something negative, only that something was intriguing and deserved investigation (some prefer to speak about enquiry-based learning). Although Dewey was not an action researcher (though he probably would have been if the term had existed then), his ideas definitely contributed to the establishment of action research as a developmental form of enquiry whose aim was to contribute to emancipatory, egalitarian and just forms of social living. He also saw living processes as evolutionary, spontaneous and context-specific, which is the view we take in this book too.

Taking these ideas into consideration, you can ask critical questions about your practice, as set out earlier on page 22:

• We review our current practice;
• identify an aspect that we want to investigate;
• imagine a way forward;
• try it out, and
• take stock of what happens.

- We modify what we are doing in light of what we find, and continue working in this way, or try another option if the new way is not right;
- monitor what we do;
- review and evaluate the modified action;
- evaluate the validity of the claim(s) to knowledge, and
- develop new practices in light of the evaluation. (See also McNiff, 2010)

It is also important that, as well as this action-focused plan, you can articulate the significance of what you are doing for others, so that they can learn from you and adopt or adapt your learning to their contexts. This highlights the need to be able to communicate effectively, through writing or other forms (Chapter 7).

You can transform these points into a series of practical questions that can then act as your action plan, as follows:

- What do I want to investigate? What is my concern?
- Why do I want to investigate it? Why am I concerned?
- What kinds of data will I gather to show the reasons for my interest/concern?
- What can I do about it? What will I do about it?
- What kinds of evidence will I generate to show the situation as it unfolds?
- How do I test the validity of my emergent claims to knowledge?
- How will I modify my concerns, ideas and practice in light of my evaluation?
- How will I explain the significance of my enquiry?

Asking questions like these can give you generic plans that may be used in different contexts and for different purposes.

> **Important!** Remember that these kinds of questions and the order in which they are presented are not fixed or static. They are not a formula. They are the kind of common-sense questions you ask to give direction to where you are going, signposts to keep you on track. You will see in this book that we ask different kinds of questions for different purposes. The main thing is to keep your eye on what you are trying to find out, and work accordingly.

Here is some practical advice for carrying out your action plan.

2. PRACTICAL ADVICE FOR CARRYING OUT YOUR ACTION PLAN

At each point, ask yourself questions about what you are doing, and consider some of the potential problematics involved.

What do I want to investigate? What is my concern?

The beginning of an action enquiry is always to ask a question of the form, 'How do I/we investigate what I am/we are doing, with a view to understanding it better, evaluating it and improving it where necessary?'. This then leads to further questions, including, 'How do I justify my actions?' and 'How do I test and demonstrate the validity of my emergent knowledge claims?'.

Remember that action research is always about taking action and doing research into that action. This works at two levels: the outer practical, in-the-world level of social action and the inner mental, in-the-head world of personal reflective action.

- You take action in the social world 'out there', by doing things differently in relation to the people you are with. You investigate what you are doing in a systematic way and keep records of your evolving activities with others.
- You take action in the personal world by thinking about what you are doing in the social world. You reflect on what you are learning, and keep records of your evolving thinking.

You learn about the action, both inner and outer, through doing the action and reflecting on what happens. Your inner and outer worlds are always in a dialectical relationship with each other, in the same way as you are always in relation with other people. Your actions are grounded in your intentionality, and, where possible, are manifestations of your values in action.

Remember also that research is about making claims to knowledge; the strongest forms of claims are those that claim to be making an original contribution to knowledge of the field. In your case, this could be knowledge about children's nursing or new forms of procedures; it can be knowledge of self and your practices with others. Remember also, from a methodological perspective, that there is a direct relationship between asking a research question (at the beginning of, say, your dissertation) and demonstrating the validity of the knowledge claims you arrive at through engaging with the question (at the end of the dissertation).

Creating a research question

From the start, aim to create a clear research question of the form 'How do I/ we ...?' or 'I wonder what would happen if I/we ...?'.

Examples of research questions are:

- How do I ensure that my technique for pre-operative care is least disturbing and most effective for patients?

- How do we evaluate the appropriateness of existing mealtime schedules to meet patients' needs?
- How do we maximise experiential learning opportunities for students in our clinical setting whilst ensuring safe practice?

You would then conduct an action enquiry to explore how to respond to these questions. Do not worry if your research question is not immediately clear. Often the question emerges as you pursue your investigations, and also the question itself may change. Your initial question, 'How do I help Mrs J to dress herself?' may turn into the more basic question, 'How do I encourage Mrs J to get out of bed?'.

Some points to note

Identifying a research issue: Aim to keep your research small, focused and manageable. Sometimes when people first start an action enquiry they ask large questions that they can do nothing about, such as 'How do we develop our organisation into a community of enquiry? How do we make the hospital more community oriented?' You can of course do this, but you can achieve more by beginning small with questions such as, 'How do I work with colleagues and patients to find ways to improve ward schedules?' or 'How can we involve community agencies in our day-to-day patient care so as to improve continuity?'.

The problematics of 'I': For the overall research community, it is still early days for the concept that 'I' is accepted as a valid actor in any enquiry. The use of 'I' in nursing research is especially problematic. Although the idea of action research is emerging in nursing research, it tends to be in a form that Torbert (2001) and Torbert and Taylor (2008) identify as 'second-person action research', within a typology of what they call first-, second- and third-person action research. Reason and Bradbury say:

> First-person action research/practice skills and methods address the ability of the researcher to foster an inquiring approach to his or her own life, to act choicefully and with awareness, and to assess effects in the outside world while acting. ... [It] provides a foundational practice and disciplines through which we can monitor the impact of our behaviour ...

> Second-person action research/practice addresses our ability to inquire face-to-face with others into issues of mutual concern – for example in the service of improving our personal and professional practice both individually and separately. Second-person inquiry starts with interpersonal dialogue and includes the development of communities of inquiry and learning organisations.

Third-person research/practice aims to extend these relatively small scale projects to create a wider impact. … third-person strategies aim to create a wider community of inquiry involving persons who, because they cannot be known to each other face-to-face … have an impersonal quality. Writing and other reporting of the process and outcomes of inquiries can also be an important form of third-person inquiry. (2008: 6)

Most second-order action research in nursing contexts still tends to take the form of an established outsider researcher, usually an academic or senior nurse, guiding the practices of clinical staff. As noted in Chapter 3, we challenge this view as ethically questionable and contradictory from the perspective of clinical nursing. As well as denying the core ethical values of acting with beneficence and care for the other and safeguarding autonomy, the positioning of one over the other tends towards the concept of authoritarian power. In this book we take the view, like Arendt (1958) that power is not a thing so much as 'the forces that constitute individuals in relation to each other' (Frazer, 2014: 156). We explore these ideas further in Chapter 9.

Why do I want to investigate this issue? Why am I concerned?

You need to be reasonably clear about why you wish to investigate this issue. For many people it may be a denial of their values in their practices, for example when they see lack of patient involvement in their own treatments or bullying behaviour on wards; or you may wish to spend more time with patients but cannot because of your workload, or find that your effort to inform a patient about a forthcoming procedure leads to distress. In every case, try to be clear about your own values position. This can be difficult because sometimes we do not understand our own motives for holding particular values. This then involves deconstructing your thinking, 'making the familiar strange'. This was an idea developed by authors such as Foucault (1980a) and Derrida (1976), where you actively distance yourself from your current thinking and try to see it through different eyes. Even then you may not get a satisfactory solution because there is also the matter of how you justify your values to yourself and others. Why do some people believe in involving patients with dementia as legitimate participants in research while others see involving them as unethical? This can lead to the interesting but disturbing dilemma where an ethical rule that was made to protect patients with dementia actually works against them by denying them the right to use their personal experience and insight to help themselves and others.

It is difficult to engage with issues like these on your own, which is where you need to talk with colleagues and patients and try to enlist their help. It is amazing how often practitioners do not see that many problematic patient-centred issues can be resolved by simply asking the patient.

What kinds of data will I gather to show the reasons for my interest/concern?

At this point you need to show what the current situation is like that you wish to investigate; this means gathering baseline data. Often when researchers begin a project they gather a good deal of data and it then becomes a matter of what Parlett and Hamilton (1977) call 'progressive focusing', when they begin actively to work with their data and more focused insights and issues emerge.

Aim to gather data according to what you are investigating, and avoid gathering irrelevant stuff. Decide what you wish to show and what kind of data will show it. Aim to gather a range of data to show the situation as it is and how it develops from different perspectives. For example, you can help a diabetic patient learn how to monitor their blood sugar levels, and you can record outcomes in a quantitative form on record charts. You can also keep records of a more qualitative nature to show how this new independence has boosted their morale, perhaps by interviewing them and/or inviting them to maintain a video diary during the process. Chapter 6 gives detailed advice about monitoring practices and gathering data. Key here is to try to gather data that is meaningful and relevant to the issue you are investigating, and make sure you keep your records up to date. It is difficult to reconstruct data after the event so aim to gather it on the spot and store it rather than leave it for another time when you will have forgotten what you did.

At a practical level you may also wish to start a blog, where you communicate with people within and beyond your workplace and solicit their advice and support. You can also use any form of social networking to post progress reports and get helpful feedback.

What can I do about it? What will I do about it?

At this point you move into action. First, look carefully at your data and begin to sort it so that themes appear (Chapter 6). Your survey results and field notes show that ward meetings are conducted by the ward manager in a quite authoritarian manner, which is leading to some clinical nurses remaining silent. Emerging themes show resentment and feelings of disempowerment among colleagues. The data show that your values of participation are being denied. What can you do?

Taking action always involves choices, all with consequences. In this case a common-sense strategy would be to talk to colleagues and ask them how they felt, and request their permission to record their responses in some way, while ensuring their anonymity if they wish. You would need also to approach the ward manager and tactfully invite their opinion about the atmosphere during meetings. You would probably write up the outcomes of the meeting as field notes or in a personal log. Trying to do something about situations like this is always delicate and calls for sensitivity and political know-how as well as courage to engage with problematic social issues. How do you tell a person that they are the problem? Inviting others to help you find strategies to tackle the issue is always useful.

What kinds of evidence will I generate to show the situation as it unfolds?

In Chapter 6 we explain the difference between data and evidence. Briefly, 'data' refers to all those pieces of information you gather that relate to your research question, and how this transforms into a knowledge claim. You gather data on an ongoing basis to show a situation as it is, how it transforms, and how the recording of the process and the results enables you to make a specific knowledge claim, such as 'I have helped diabetic patients learn how to control their blood sugar levels' or 'I have contributed to the development of more democratic ward meetings'. 'Evidence' refers to those particular pieces of data that show in action the criteria you identify to make judgements about what is happening (Chapter 6).

How do I test the validity of my emergent claims to knowledge?

The matter of testing the validity of knowledge claims is dealt with in detail in Chapter 7. Briefly, it refers to the idea that you do not expect people to believe your claims without giving them good reason in the form of authenticated evidence that grounds your claims. Your claim that you have helped diabetic patients is grounded in evidence, authenticated by the patients themselves, to show that you really have helped them. Testing validity like this enables you to show that you have acted responsibly by making your research available for public scrutiny, and have acted on the feedback of critical peers, including patients. You have gone through rigorous professional and academic procedures such as establishing a validation group that meets periodically to review your research findings and offers critical feedback. You can show that you have acted on the feedback, and the processes involved.

How will I modify my concerns, ideas and practice in light of my evaluation?

When you do action research you are also carrying out a form of evaluation. There are different kinds of evaluation, including formative evaluation and summative evaluation. Formative evaluation refers to ongoing assessment, which enables you to give progress reports and identify what is going well and what still needs to be done; summative evaluation is carried out at the end of a particular phase of the enquiry. You can also conduct a personal evaluation of your own practice, and invite others to conduct an objective evaluation. All these strategies are valuable, because they show that you are serious about testing the validity of your knowledge claim, coming at it from multiple directions, and revising it as appropriate. For example, you may find that a validation group disagrees that you have helped diabetic patients, because some patients said that they still could not control their blood sugar levels. It would then be important to establish why this was the case by talking with the patients in question. However, if you get positive feedback, and feel that things are moving in the right direction, you will probably continue working in this way, while constantly evaluating what you are doing and recording the processes involved.

How will I explain the significance of my research?

Explaining the significance of your research means you are able to give cogent explanations for what you have done – that is, you can give reasons and purposes for the research, and also say how you have addressed them. You can explain and analyse why it is important to have done the research and who will benefit from your new knowledge: you are able to reflect on your analyses and explanations, and say why they are important and who they are important for. A useful way of recording these matters is to show the movement from description to analytic reflection through your journal, as in Table 5.1.

Here is a real-life example to show the action plan in action.

Table 5.1 Reflective diary: from description to analysis

What I did	I talked with Mr Brooks, a diabetic patient, and showed him how he could control his blood sugar levels.
Why I did it	I did this because I believe that it is important for all people, including diabetic patients, to be in control of their own lives. This allows people an increased sense of autonomy and independence.
What I learned from what I did	I learned how to explain these matters to diabetic patients. From Mr Brooks's responses I learned more about the importance for diabetic patients of being in control of their own bodies. I learned about some of the day-to-day complications that make it difficult to follow care regimes.
The significance of my actions and my learning	The significance of my actions and my learning is that I now know more about helping diabetic patients than I knew before. I have also learned the importance of making my knowledge public so that other nurse colleagues can adapt these ideas to their own practices if they wish. In this way I have contributed to new forms of thinking and practice for practising nurses through doing my action research. Perhaps professional bodies will take seriously the idea that clinical nurses can research their own practices and contribute valuable knowledge for the advancement of the profession.

3. EXAMPLE OF AN ACTION PLAN IN ACTION: IMPROVING PLACEMENTS FOR NEW NURSES

Here is the story of an action enquiry.

What do I want to investigate?

I am a clinical manager in a busy medical unit with 24 patients (beds) and a high occupancy rate. An ongoing issue for our ward staff is how to help new staff who come onto the unit, including a number of students on placement, to learn how to fit into our work pattern and contribute to the everyday work as quickly as possible. This is important because everyone needs to work together to ensure patients get effective treatment speedily and efficiently. Our student placements are supported primarily by the university education liaison service, but we are still largely responsible for their education in the clinical area. This as an important element of our work but it is also time consuming and difficult to prioritise at particularly busy times. When newly qualified staff or students arrive with us we often find that their clinical skills are under-developed and they are of course not familiar with our work patterns. Helping them get used to how we work means we have to take time out that we should be spending elsewhere, especially with patients. But due to chronic staffing shortages these new staff are effectively regarded as part of the existing workforce and no allowance is made for their lack of contribution at this point. Many of them go on to develop into excellent clinical nurses, but to help them do this means that we have to find ways of creating a work pattern that has a more seamless link between our actual work and the education and training of the new staff.

Why do I want to investigate it?

It is really important that we investigate this and try to find a better way of doing things because there is no spare capacity in our staffing levels. Also, because of shift patterns, there is little overlap time or down time which in the past we may have used to do extra education and training for all staff. At present new staff do not contribute much in their early stages and also take up more of the time and attention of established staff while going through this steep early learning phase. Although we have made the case to hospital management that it would genuinely be much more efficient to build in capacity to train and develop people and therefore get them up to speed more quickly this case has never been accepted.

What kinds of data will I gather to show the reasons for my concern?

When time has allowed (no extra time has been built in to our system to allow for any research and is not likely to be), we have collected data during routine interviews with staff and have recorded these as ward notes. We try to have these interviews on a regular basis to identify any problems experienced individually or as a team. The issue of getting new staff quickly up to speed has been highlighted spontaneously by a number of colleagues, so a good deal of anecdotal and interview data is available, usually recorded as field notes or in diary jottings, to show that this is a real problem that affects a lot of people. I have kept my own log, which I make available to anyone who wishes to see it, including patients. Second, we asked key members of staff to maintain a simple record of their activities, i.e. what they were doing at a specific point in time, and asked them to fill it in every half hour. This highlighted the fact that when a new member of staff had been placed in a team the amount of time spent in advising, demonstrating and training was increased.

What can I do about it? What will I do about it?

We have in a sense already taken action in identifying this as an urgent issue, as part of the regular staff meetings we hold to allow time for staff to discuss issues and raise items relevant to their work and the smooth running of the unit. Both experienced and new staff indicated that this was a matter of priority. We therefore decided to do some serious on-the-spot research to clarify the issue and help us to find ways of improving this situation. We also felt that if we could make an evidence-based case for developing new forms of induction for new staff we could perhaps persuade management to work with us to look at more realistic staffing levels. We hoped that an evidenced outcome of our research would make a realistic case for more staff.

We did not have any clear set procedure or precedent that we could identify as the basis for a particular research approach, so partly for this reason we decided that an action research approach would be most effective. Another reason for this decision was that action research lends itself to being carried out in the workplace during work time by practice-based staff and is therefore less time diverting than calling in an external researcher who might use time-consuming data gathering methods. We used some of the time available for handovers and discussions to decide how to conduct our action research and had free discussions where colleagues could put forward suggestions for consideration by everyone about whether these would be worth trying. We also invited the university-based education department to meet with us to see what contribution they could make. They said that they would wish to be supportive but that much of their time was focused on meeting the demands of the curriculum and they had no spare capacity to increase time in the clinical area.

So we decided that a first approach would be to identify a number of common themes that regularly crop up as problematic for new members of staff. All members of staff helped to draw up a list of areas that arose on almost every occasion. This gave us a working brief as to how we could prepare our own clinical-based system of introduction and training, obviously in addition to the standard induction already mandated by hospital managers. We then held discussions between experienced and new staff, many sharing their own experiences, about what would be the best way to make this learning available to new people. We compiled a number of worksheets that gave advice and information about the items we had identified as being problematic and agreed that these would be issued to new staff prior to their coming to work in our clinical area. They would then be allocated a key team member who would act as their mentor and each would agree to spend a short period each day discussing any items arising.

How will I keep track of everything? What kind of data can I gather to show the situation as it unfolds?

We agreed that it would be the responsibility of the new member of staff to keep their own record of learning, to be filled out at the end of the day, along with a record of their discussions with their mentor. This would include actions to be taken and the results of those actions when carried out. This then provided a written record of developments and indicated where improvements were taking place as well as being an early warning system for issues arising. In addition to this, as the clinical manager with overall responsibility, I met regularly, albeit briefly, with each new member of staff to discuss progress. I asked them to be responsible for keeping a record of these meetings. This gave them responsibility and leadership in developing their own learning as part of the team but ensured that it reflected the point of view of the whole team rather than being seen only as the individual engaged in self-directed learning. Our ongoing ward staff discussions provided verbal data of improvements in the area we were investigating, and staff indicated that the transition of new staff to levels of greater experience was easier. It also became noticeable that all staff became more enthusiastic about the project as it developed and began to take on a life of its own.

How will I test the validity of my claims to knowledge?

We identified criteria to help us transform our data into evidence. These took the form of the needs and values we had specified as the basis of improving our work situation – that is, that new staff had to learn the job as quickly as possible, and that transitions from novice to more competent nursing (Benner, 1984) could be effected as smoothly as possible. We appreciated that all our data stood as valid qualitative evidence as it is realistic and practice-based, although it would be judged as somewhat unmeasurable by conventional research methods.

How will I ensure that any conclusions I reach are reasonably fair and accurate?

We scheduled brief meetings to keep track of what we were doing. We thought about inviting patients to these meetings, but decided against it as the focus of the enquiry was a specific issue of staffing. During the meetings we attempted to triangulate our observations and data. This meant that, having already gathered the views of newly inducted staff, university-based education staff and our own clinical area workers, when we returned after experimenting with new induction systems we were able to obtain multiple viewpoints of effects and changes. Feedback was varied: some people saw our experiment as working, while others made suggestions about how we could tighten up procedures and develop new strategies. Many lively and good-natured discussions took place, from which many people said they learned a great deal.

How will I modify my concerns, ideas and practice in light of my evaluation?

We were encouraged by our university-based colleagues to think of our research as a way in which we were developing new theories, generated by our studies into our practices. In our case, these would be theories of collaborative working and developing a culture of learning. It had become clear to us that we were all learning collectively and that we were able to articulate our learning in explicit terms, which we had never done before. A key point here was that our learning had great significance for us both at individual levels and also for the smooth running of the unit, which raised our personal learning to systemic levels. We could say that we were contributing to organisational learning.

How will I communicate the significance of my claims to knowledge?

We agreed to write this experiment up as a piece of practice-based research, as led by the clinical team and that addressed an identified problem. We offered our report to be disseminated to other clinical areas, although we made no claims for generalisability or replicability other than that people could perceive the relevance of what we had learned for their own practices and theories and try similar things out for themselves. We felt that the information contained would be useful to people facing similar real-life problems.

The significance is that this enabled us to carry out some genuinely helpful research without hugely adding to our workload or introducing outside elements which would often be intrusive and time consuming. It allowed a team approach to solving a problem arising in our own clinical area, using a methodology that lent itself to a busy working situation.

4. DRAWING UP A SCHEDULE FOR AN ACTION ENQUIRY

Finally, draw up a schedule for your own action enquiry (see Table 5.2). This enables you to combine the practical, logistical and organisational matters outlined in Chapter 4 and the methodological issues outlined in this chapter. The notional schedule in Table 5.2 is for a three-month project, which is fairly typical of a CPD course or a Masters module. It is meant to show how to draw up a schedule: you should supply information as per your own work and time circumstances.

So now, all you need to do is to do it.

Table 5.2 Notional schedule for an action research project

Task undertaken	Time completed
Planning and preparation	
• Identify research area and research issue	Week 1
• Initial reading and literature search	Weeks 2-6
• Plan and design project	Week 2-3
• Identification of topic and research question	Week 3
• Draw up ethics statements	Weeks 3-4
• Application to ethics committee	Weeks 3-4
• Convene collaborative group of critical friends as project advisors	Weeks 3-4
Resourcing	
• Draw up budget	Week 3
• Submit request for funding	Week 3
• Negotiate availability of videocamera	Week 4
• Negotiate availability of multimedia room for interviews	Week 4
Working with others	
• Discussions with management and policy makers	Week 3
• Invitations to potential participants	Weeks 2-4
• Invitation to critical friends	Weeks 2-4

Task undertaken	Time completed
• Invitation to potential validation group	Weeks 2-4
• Distribution of letters confirming ethical conduct, as consent is given	Weeks 2-4
• Initiation of blog and project website	Week 2

Doing the project

• Identify research issue/concern: check with others	Week 3
• Articulate research question	Week 3
• Review overall situation; stocktaking exercise; explain why the situation needs investigating	Weeks 3-4
• Data gathering, first round	Weeks 3-4
• Identify working criteria and standards of judgement	Weeks 3-4
• First meeting of validation group; formative assessment	Week 5
• Imagining solutions; brainstorming with colleagues and patients	Weeks 4-5
• Try out possible actions; take stock of outcomes	Weeks 3-6
• Regular meetings with critical friends	Weeks 2-7
• Data gathering, second round, and later rounds as appropriate	Weeks 4-7
• Data analysis and interpretation; coding and categorising; generating evidence	Weeks 5-7
• Second meeting of validation group; formative assessment	Weeks 5-6
• Articulate knowledge claim and test its validity through specific validation procedures	Weeks 5-6
• Articulate the significance of the project and findings	Weeks 8-9
• Final meeting of validation group; summative assessment	Week 10

Evaluating the significance of the project

• Produce working project report	Weeks 6-8
• Explain significance of own learning	Weeks 7-8
• Explain significance of the project for others' learning	Weeks 7-8

Writing up the project report

• Draft report produced and disseminated to participants and interested colleagues; critical feedback invited	Weeks 8-9
• Final report produced and disseminated to participants and interested colleagues	Week 12

Dissemination of findings

• Planning for dissemination	Weeks 8-9
• Action plan for production of further reports	Weeks 8-9
• Action plan for production of conference papers and conferences to be attended	Weeks 11-12
• Action plan for convening special interest group in workplace	Weeks 11-12

SUMMARY

This chapter has outlined how to draw up and carry out action plans. It has given advice about different approaches and models and how these might be realised in practice. Practical advice is given for different steps in an action enquiry, at different levels of progress. An example of an action plan is provided. Finally, a framework for drawing up a timetable or schedule for conducting an action enquiry is offered.

Reflective questions

- Outline some of the models you have read about for drawing up an action plan.
- What do you think might be some of the problematics involved in carrying out an action enquiry? Is it all straightforward? Do you need to get it absolutely right?
- What practical advice would you give to a colleague who is planning to conduct an action enquiry?
- Why do you think it is important to maintain a reflective journal?
- Draw up your own schedule for an action enquiry. Do you think you will stick to your timetable? Have you left wiggle room for unforeseen circumstances?

SIX

Monitoring practices and gathering data

This chapter is about monitoring your practices and gathering useful and relevant data. This means thinking about what you are looking for and where and how you might find it. It involves decisions about how you are going to monitor and keep track of what you are doing, including changes in your thinking and learning. This is important, because everything you do potentially influences what other people do and you need to keep a record of the processes involved.

Gathering data is multifaceted and complex. Life and practices are seldom straightforward, so gathering, interpreting and analysing data will probably also not be straightforward. You need to engage with the complexity and show how you have made sense out of a dynamic and possibly problematic situation.

In your action research you ask the following questions:

1. Which data do I look for? Data about what?
2. How do I gather data? Which data gathering methods do I use?
3. When and where do I gather data?
4. How do I manage the data? How do I sort and store it?

The chapter is organised to address these questions.

A note on our terminology: Some people say 'data is' and some say 'data are'. Both forms are in common use though technically 'data are' is the correct form, translated from Latin. In this book we tend to use both forms as best suits the context.

1. WHICH DATA DO I LOOK FOR? DATA ABOUT WHAT?

You conduct your research in order to engage with a research question with a view to making a claim to knowledge, which, if possible, will constitute an original contribution to knowledge of the field; in your case, knowledge of nursing practices. Whatever you look for will be in relation to your research question. There is always a direct link between your research question and your knowledge claim. You ask at the beginning of your project, 'How do I help this patient?' and you say at the end of the project, 'I have helped this patient and I can describe and explain how and why I have done so'. You can also analyse the significance of what you have done. Showing this relationship between question and claim enables you to show the methodological rigour of your research: all the pieces fit together coherently as you trace your pathway from question to claim. The story of Theseus and the Minotaur can help: when Theseus went to find the Minotaur he had to find his way through a maze. The goddess Ariadne gave him a golden thread to tie to the gatepost and unwind as he went. He could then retrace his steps back to the gate by following the golden thread. The same golden thread runs through your research. When you write your report or dissertation, you put your claim at the beginning of the text to explain to your reader what you have achieved, and you spend the rest of the text showing how you came to make the claim and how you have tested its validity (believability) (see Chapter 8).

The word 'data' refers to all those pieces of information that show how you are engaging with your research question, so you need always to keep your research question in mind as your lodestar. You can appear to take a circuitous route occasionally but your research question brings you back on track and makes sure you stay there.

As a nurse-researcher you work with two interrelated and inseparable questions, one about your actions and the other about your research.

- Your action-oriented question tends to take the form: 'How do I help this person?' and you gather data to show what you are doing. Your actions are always in relation with other people, so you also gather data about how your actions are influencing them.
- Your research-oriented question tends to take the form: 'How do I learn to help this person more effectively?' This kind of question is about your learning, where you systematically investigate what you are doing so that you can evaluate it and improve it according to what you find out. You gather data about these processes too.

In action research the two questions always go together because learning takes place in and emerges from your action, and informs future actions in an ongoing cyclical process. Actions and learning are always interrelated. You try to improve your learning so that you can develop better, more informed actions.

Your learning also has the potential to influence other people's learning, which they can use to inform their new actions. This emphasises the educational nature of action research. You and they are in a reciprocal transformational relationship where your collective learning becomes a self-regenerating exponential system, with infinite potential for influencing new learning and new actions. So when you look for data you look for those episodes that show the transformational interactions between yourself and others with whom you are in contact, as set out in Figure 6.1.

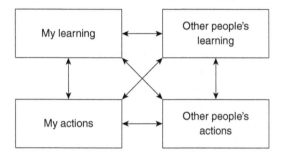

Figure 6.1 Reciprocal transformational relationships between personal and social action and learning (adapted from McNiff, 2016)

Some points to note are:

- Your research is always informed by your values; you carry out your research in order to find ways of living your values in your practices. The kinds of values that inform nursing are to do with personal empathy, interactive skills and holistic understanding and effectiveness for patients' wellbeing. Your research question will always be something about how you can realise your values in practice, and if not, how you can overcome whatever is stopping you. As an individual you ask, 'How do I encourage my colleagues to develop successful team nursing?'. As a collective you ask, 'How do we develop successful team nursing?'.
- Action research questions tend to engage with the underlying question, 'How do I understand, evaluate and improve my practices where necessary?', from the implicit commitment to living in the direction of your values. Your practices take place both in the head, when you are thinking, and in the social situation, when you are in company with other people. Even if you are not in direct physical contact with them, you are still connected through relationships of influence over space and time.
- Developing understanding, evaluating and improving something happens over time, so you will need to track your actions and learning as they happen and keep records before you forget. Interpreting also happens over time, so it is important to keep records of your interpretations, because these will inevitably give way to new interpretations and new understandings.
- Practices and learning do not 'just happen'. Actions can 'just happen', such as laughing or tripping over, but these are actions and not practices. Practices are always informed, committed and intentional. What you are looking for in your data, therefore, is what you knew at a particular time, and how this transformed into new knowledge over time, so that you came to a point where you knew something that you did not know before, or that you came to know it better. Ideally you are looking for episodes where you took informed, committed and intentional action. The idea of informed, committed and intentional action

gives us the concept of praxis. As a clinical nurse you always aim to engage in praxis; you always try to show what it means to embody the wisdom of care.

Also remember that gathering data is just the first piece of a quite complex process that involves three distinct operations:

1. Collecting data in order to give a clear description about what you and others are doing (outlined in this chapter).
2. Interpreting and analysing the data you have collected so that you can begin to explain what you are doing (outlined in Chapter 7).
3. Evaluating what you are doing so that you can show its educational value, and so continue with the action or re-plan in light of your evaluation (also outlined in Chapter 7).

Here are the different aspects you (ideally) need to gather data about, as set out in Figure 6.1:

- your learning;
- your actions;
- other people's learning;
- other people's actions.

Monitoring your learning and gathering data about it

Here are some ways in which you can gather data about how your learning is developing. These tend to be from (a) other people's feedback and (b) your own reflections.

Other people's feedback can be quite straightforward, as when they send you an email or text message saying, 'I really enjoyed what you said in the meeting. It is clear to me that you appreciate the situation much better than before, and probably have a better grasp of it now than anyone else on the committee'. You would expect your supervisor or professional mentor to write these kinds of notes as comments on your assignments, or perhaps your colleague could write you a note for inclusion in your performance review.

Possibly the most effective and powerful form of monitoring your own learning and gathering data about it is through a reflective journal. More is said about this below, but just to note that a journal or diary can take the form of a traditional paper journal, or a diary that you keep on your computer, or perhaps following a thread through emails or social networking. You can keep a record of correspondence with others that shows how they are commenting on your learning, and you on theirs, and you can also keep a record of your own reflections on your learning. Your data shows the process of rethinking assumptions, and then rethinking your earlier rethinking. This can be especially effective because it shows the process of transformative learning, a process developed by several researchers including:

- Jack Mezirow, who describes it as 'the process by which adults learn how to think critically for themselves rather than take assumptions supporting a point of view for granted' (2009: 103); and
- Stephen Brookfield, who comments that 'The ability to be critically analytical concerning the assumptions underlying our own actions and those of others is organizationally and culturally beneficial as well as personally liberating' (1987: 43). It can also, however, be personally destabilising, when you critique assumptions that you have held all your life and suddenly come to see that they did not serve you well.

By monitoring your learning in this way you are able to use your reflective journal entries as data that show the processes involved in your learning and your re-learning, and the significance of the process. Schön and Rein (1994) speak of this process as 'reframing', when you rethink past assumptions, and then rethink your rethinking. Most portfolio records work like this, where you collect instances of performance at particular points in your work life, and provide a commentary on the value and potential significance of what you have done and achieved. Doing this enables you to offer explanations for your learning and how it informs your actions (you are able to theorise what you are doing) and also articulate the significance of your learning for future actions.

Monitoring your actions and gathering data about them

You can monitor your actions and gather data about them yourself, or you can ask other people to help you. You are looking for data that relate specifically to your research question. If your question is, 'How do I help Mrs Smith to become more self-motivating in her rehabilitation exercises?' you will look for data that show you encouraging and helping Mrs Smith to do her rehabilitation exercises. Remember that research questions are always linked with values. You are probably helping Mrs Smith to do her exercises because you hold values around people's wellbeing and the fact that they should be able to move about properly. You therefore not only look for data that show you helping her do her exercises, from a functional perspective, but that also show whether the exercises contribute to her sense of wellbeing, from a holistic, engaged perspective. Your actions are always informed by your commitment to certain values. This involves ethical choices, whether you act in your own interests or other people's. You would ask Mrs Smith whether you had helped her to do her exercises more regularly, and whether she felt this was doing her good. She could give you her responses in a range of ways: she could write you a note, or send you an email.

Remember that actions are never taken in isolation in social contexts; they are always related to other people. This is especially the case in nursing practices, where you work for the benefit of others. As with Mrs Smith, you would seek feedback from the people you are trying to help, to see if you are succeeding or not. You could try the following strategies:

- Ask patients to keep records and make a note of the situation at regular times and give feedback.
- Ask an individual member of staff to make observations on a regular basis and show you their records.
- Issue a questionnaire for patients or staff asking them about how they experience your work with them.

You would also keep your own records of practice and your reflections on them, probably through a personal journal. Some nurses maintain a video diary where they record their actions and reflections, and some maintain a blog or social networking site, where they share their accounts with others. Many practitioners write up their informal notes as emails or tweets. These can also act as records of your learning and show changes in your attitudes, beliefs and knowledge, which indicates that growth and learning are taking place. At a more formal level, you would keep daily records of practice after each meaningful interaction with a patient, which would be available for other colleagues to see.

Monitoring other people's learning and gathering data about it

It is questionable whether you can monitor other people's learning because learning is an individual experience that goes on inside people's heads. Only learners can say what they are learning. You can definitely make judgements about people's learning from listening to them or from reading their texts. You can hear or read their accounts of the process of their learning, and see the outcomes in social spaces.

You can also request access to people's learning journals, to see how their learning takes place. They would keep reflective journals in the same way as you do, to keep a record of their learning and actions to show how both are developing.

Susan works with student nurses on a paediatric ward. She wants to see how they are learning to work with children and families, taking into account their medical, social, cultural and family circumstances. She believes strongly in the power of group work, where individuals challenge one another's assumptions and help them find ways to challenge their own. She invites the student nurses to maintain records of their learning, in diaries and through assignments. She maintains her own reflective diary, which she makes available to the student nurses. Those records show how, as a group that includes Susan, they negotiated their learning together and achieved a higher state of reflection and knowledge.

As in this example, it is important to monitor what happens in social interactions that enable people to learn, and to see what happens when they do. It is especially important in the kind of dialogical relationships we are recommending in this book, where nurses, patients, colleagues and families work together with the common goal of moving towards full engagement in life and a sense of wellbeing for all.

A strong literature exists to support this view. Freire (1970) believed that communication is the basis of how we create and recreate ourselves, in negotiation with others. He spoke about dialogic action, when people decide to take action together, a theme developed by Habermas (1976) who emphasised the need for authentic communication in order to take action. Bakhtin (1986) specifically noted that learning can be understood as a social practice, and Seely Brown and Duguid (2000) note that you can learn as much over the photocopier or coffee cups as when attending a formal lecture. This theme has been developed vigorously in nursing practices by Benner (1984) and Benner et al. (2010) who call for a dialogical approach in nursing education, as do Binnie and Titchen (1999), Higgs and Titchen (2001) and others. This point is especially important for nurses since nursing is an eminently social, in-the-moment practice, always conducted with and assessed by others.

Monitoring other people's actions and gathering data about them

It is reasonably straightforward to monitor other people's actions and gather data about them through simple observation and recording what is going on. You can compare what happens today with what happened a week ago and show progress, or not as the case may be.

It is important, however, to remember how you position yourself in your research. In conventional forms of social science research you position yourself as an outsider who is observing others and making judgements about what they are doing. In action research you position yourself as an insider who is working with others in a dialogical way, so you do not make judgements about what they are doing so much as what you are doing to help them work or respond in particular ways, and therefore what you do collectively.

Also remember that contextual issues can have a major bearing on how people act.

For example, you could be the primary nurse who is in charge of admitting a patient with acute fever of unknown origin. You know that the patient has recently returned from a visit to a tropical country. While official diagnosis would be a doctor's responsibility it is your responsibility to put in place a system of care that ensures

(Continued)

(Continued)

the wellbeing of the patient while protecting staff and others from the spread of any possible infection. You therefore gather data from the patient themselves and their family about their recent activities to build up a picture of the context. You liaise with the admitting doctor to see what the most likely outcomes might be, and inform the path lab of the likelihood of specimens coming down which you would like prioritised. It may be helpful to have an initial consultation with the infection control nurse to indicate the level of precautions necessary, which you record, and to contact any staff who are familiar with the country from which the patient has returned for any information they may be able to give. You use all these data to help you make decisions about priorities for care and possible preventive measures.

2. HOW DO I GATHER DATA? WHICH DATA GATHERING METHODS DO I USE?

You can gather data using a range of data-gathering techniques or methods, some of which are listed below. There are no strict guidelines about which methods to use for which data. It is up to you to decide which method best suits your purposes, so use your common sense and sensitivity about the choices you make. Ask yourself:

- How do I gather data? What techniques are available?
- Where and when do I gather data?

How do I gather data? What techniques are available?

A range of protocols is available in the literatures about how to gather data using different techniques and strategies. To a certain extent this depends on whether you decide to gather quantitative or qualitative forms of data. Some texts state that you can use only qualitative forms in action research, which is not the case. For example, you can definitely record quantitatively a patient's fluid balance on their fluid balance chart, which would give you important feedback about what kind of actions you should take. Be aware, however, that in nursing a lot of changes can be quite subtle, and would require more meaningful, often values-oriented, information that is not restricted simply to quantitative methods.

One of the most useful protocols comes from Creswell (2007: 130), who organises data collection approaches as:

- observations;
- interviews;

- documents;
- audiovisual and multimedia materials and performances.

Using this typology, consider the different methods available.

Observations: field notes

All data gathering begins with observation. You watch what is going on for yourself and others, and keep track of it in some way. Elliott (1991) speaks about the first phases of an action enquiry as including a reconnaissance phase during which you take stock of what is happening.

You can make field notes as you carry out your enquiry. These can be informal jottings on paper, iPad or smartphone, on the back of your hand, or any other way of keeping a record. Gather your field notes about what you observe in the field, and also about what is going on in your thinking. Carry a notepad or recording device with you all the time (your smartphone will do) to keep a record of observations, new ideas and what you are reading at the time. You can also use your smartphone to take photos or videos of interactions, and add a commentary to note the significance of what is happening, or to link it with the literatures you are reading or a commentary from this week's nursing newsletter. Remember to get permission from the participant and ethics committee if you wish to use your video recordings.

Different forms of graphic representation can be useful – for example, concept maps or spider diagrams, which follow much the same process as tracking and linking ideas. You can also monitor and record social interactions using simple interaction charts, such as shown in Figure 6.2.

	half-hour intervals			
	12.30–13.00	13.01– 13.30	13.31–14.00	14.01–14.30
Number of patient–nurse interactions	I	JHT	IIII	I

Figure 6.2 Record sheet to show number of interactions between patient and nurse

You can gather field notes about yourself or other people, from an outsider or insider perspective. You can make field notes about you and other people or you can ask other people to make field notes about you. You would transcribe and tidy up these notes as soon as possible after the event so that they are fresh in your memory.

Interviews

Interviews are used extensively in action research to obtain information from participants about their opinions and experiences. They are often equivalent to live surveys and can take several forms:

- Structured interviews where you ask your participant specific open-ended questions and take notes or record the interview. Use a questionnaire to ask closed questions where you are looking for specific answers.
- Semi-structured interviews, where you ask specific questions but invite the participant to give more extensive answers, and record or keep notes.
- Focus group interviews, where you record or ask an observer to keep notes.
- Electronic interviews, using computers or other devices for text messages and emails. These can be audio or visual, telephone and online using web links or interactive messaging.

In all interviews remember that you or someone else can keep notes, and written and recorded notes need to be transcribed afterwards. Be careful about ethical issues when interviewing. Important points to note are:

- Pilot the interview before doing it live. Practise your interviewing skills with a colleague and get their feedback about your performance.
- Negotiate to record the interview. Never record without asking permission.
- Tell your interviewee what the interview is about and check if they agree. Tell them if you cannot tell them what it is about. Give them whatever information they need.
- Be prepared to listen more than you speak. Learn to accept silences. Demonstrate empathy and be patient.
- Don't mislead or deceive people into giving you information.
- Always give your transcripts back to your participants for them to check, and negotiate the final document with them so that they are comfortable with what you have produced.
- Never use any transcript data without permission. This will lose participants' trust, which you will never be able to regain.
- Be honorable at all times.

Documentary data

Documents take a range of forms, including the following.

Logs, diaries and journals

Aim to keep a diary throughout your research and ask your participants to do the same. Diaries can take the form of conventional written notes – on paper or electronically – and take the form of drawings or symbolic representations. They can also appear as a thread of emails, texts or other forms of messaging devices. You can also keep video diaries, which can give you comprehensive documentary evidence of progress.

Diaries help you to do the following:

- You can keep a record of daily activities. Aim to write up your diary as soon as possible after the event. Especially keep a note of any specific comments you or others make.
- They help you to reflect on experience and evaluate it, and to rethink and interrogate your own thinking where appropriate. Ongoing reflection can help you rethink the rethinking, which is essential in any kind of professional education programme.
- They help to keep you on track, by showing alerts and 'to do' lists. Diaries can also give you a timeline and storyline for your research when you write it up.
- You can invite participants to keep reflective journals, and ask if you may see them, but be prepared for people to refuse. Journals can be sensitive documents. If other people's journals are essential to your research, negotiate access in advance.
- **NB:** Never use participants' comments or diary entries without permission. Doing so will lose their trust, which you will never regain. Be warned.

Letters and correspondence

Keep records of important and relevant documents and correspondence, in particular:

- Keep records of who said what, when and why; this gives you a trail that helps you monitor the process of your research, keep a record of events, and make sure you stay on track.
- Minutes and agendas similarly help you to keep a record and stay on track.
- Work out a filing system for keeping your own records; perhaps keep a loose-leaf file or computer file that you can rearrange as necessary, and make sure you consult it regularly. You can use sticky notes on your computer desktop or any kind of productivity app on your electronic device.

Public documents and records

Public documents and records are important for recording current and past practices, and can include institutional archives, agendas and minutes of meetings and policy statements. They can be helpful for providing contextual issues for your studies. For example, *Nursing Times* and RCN documents provide important factual information about past and current developments in the field. You would use these records for establishing what was going on in the situation you were investigating and any social or political forces that were helping or hindering you in your enquiry. Accessing and looking at records is often called 'desk research' or 'library research'.

Audiovisual and multimedia materials and performances

These are used increasingly in formal action research accounts and take the form of videotaped and multimedia recordings. They show the live realities of practices and interactions, including the responses of others to what is said and done, so they capture live meanings more effectively than written texts.

Most higher education institutions now accept multimedia as evidence of professional development and learning. They also accept live music, dance and artwork performances, as well as videotaped recordings of these. Many online journals also accept multimedia representations, though these would also be framed using a linguistic form that outlines how they were constructed and what their significance is for the field. Butler-Kisber (2010) identifies different forms of performance: poetic inquiry, collage inquiry, photographic inquiry and performative inquiry. She comments:

> [Performative inquiry] offers an important lens for thinking about inquiry that is embodied, relational, participatory, and geared to action and social change. Promise lies in the continued exploration of this form of inquiry. (2010: 146)

The following comment is especially relevant to clinical nursing practices:

> … to retain and develop more fully an ethical stance in all aspects of research, there needs to be an upfront and continuous questioning of the 'so what' or utility of our work. Does our work make a difference, and if so for whom, and how and why? These kinds of discussions cannot remain relegated to scholarly circles in academe. They must reach the public domain in ways that are accessible, informative, and engaging. (Butler-Kisber, 2010: 150)

3. WHEN DO I GATHER DATA?

To a certain extent you need to be entrepreneurial in data gathering and watch out for opportunities. You should aim to gather data at every point of your action enquiry. Here is a notional outline of how you can do this. We take a simplified form of an action enquiry to illustrate these ideas.

What do I wish to investigate? What is my concern?

Identify the focus of your enquiry and keep a record in your notebook or written or video diary. Make sure you date every entry so you can keep a chronological record, which is important in watching how your actions and thinking change over time. Historical accounts can provide important sources of data.

Why do I wish to investigate this issue? Why is it a concern?

- You could videotape a conversation between yourself and a colleague when you speak about your values and what gives meaning to your life, and refer to these when you speak about why you wish to do the research. This tape can act as a baseline document, to show the genesis of your enquiry.
- You can find documentary evidence in private and public documents to show how your values are being denied in your practice.
- You read about your area of enquiry and keep notes in your learning journal. You identify key conceptual frameworks for your research. Make sure you keep your references, especially page references for any quotations. Keep a list of references on your computer and update it regularly.

How do I show the situation as it is and the reasons for my concern?

- Search public records and media reports to show contextual issues in action.
- Interview participants to solicit their feedback about the issue you are investigating.
- Maintain field notes as you observe people in the kind of situation you are investigating.

What do I do? What actions do I take?

- Keep a daily diary of events. Make sure you date everything accurately. Ask participants to do the same.
- Interview others to get their feedback on dilemmas and problematic situations. Ask their advice.
- Write a letter to networks outlining your research question and ask for feedback and advice about how to tackle it. Do the same using social media and blogs. Keep a record of responses and date each one.

How do I generate evidence to show how the situation unfolds?

- Tape-record a conversation with a critical friend about how you intend to search your data archive. Discuss which themes you could identify as guiding principles.
- Produce a contents list of your data archive. Make sure all entries are dated and original documents signed as appropriate. Make photocopies of paper documents for inclusion as appendices in official research reports.

- Keep an archive of videotapes that show participants discussing ideas relevant to your issue. Select from the archive those pieces that show changes in thinking, and write a contextualising summary to show how this happened.

How do I ensure that any conclusions I come to are reasonably fair and accurate?

- Video record a validation meeting to show how you invited critical responses from your validation group on your provisional knowledge claims.
- Keep a record of the documentation you submitted for their scrutiny.
- Write to your networks to review where you are in your research, and indicate any new directions following their feedback.

How do I modify my ideas and practices in light of my evaluation?

- Use any kind of data recording device to show how you and others are developing new individual and collective practices.
- Hold a videotaped conversation with the same colleague as at the beginning of your research, to comment on its history and potential significance.
- Do a videotaped seminar for staff who may be interested in learning about your research and its potentials for organisational learning.

Now think about how you are going to manage the data.

4. HOW DO I MANAGE THE DATA? HOW DO I SORT AND STORE IT?

It is important to manage your data effectively, to save you time and energy when you are trying to locate a specific item. You can do this using traditional printed paper methods, though it is increasingly common to organise data electronically to save space and cut down on paper usage. Most higher education institutions offer advice on how you can manage your data, sort it and retrieve it and many helpful tutorials are available online. Type in 'organising and managing data' to your search engine and you will find lots of advice from different institutions: for example, see www.york.ac.uk/library/info-for/researchers/data/organising/#tab-4 for one of the best. If you are working with others or as a team, negotiate how you are going to store information and how you will name different aspects. It is important to have these common agreements to save time and effort and avoid unnecessary delays in processing information.

The most common advice offered for sorting and storing data is as follows:

- Categorise your data according to themes and headings: for example, 'conversations' or 'interviews'. You can refine these categories to help you to search for specific items – for example, 'Conversations with colleagues; conversations with patients'. Be confident about which labels you choose and be consistent from the start. Also organise your photos and videos using the same organising principles. Categorising is essential when it comes to analysing and interpreting your data with a view to generating evidence (Chapter 7).
- Name files and folders according to subject matter ('Feedback from patients') or persons ('Conversations with Jo') or events ('Graduation day 2015'). Use whatever system is best for you. Helpful advice is given in the Jisc Digital Media Guide at www.jiscdigitalmedia.ac.uk/guide/choosing-a-file-name
- Always give a file a date. This helps you locate your files across time.
- Create folders where you can store files, and label the folders accurately. Once you have named a folder do not then give it another name unless absolutely necessary. We tend to remember the first name we give to something.
- Keep your files and folders active. Constantly revisit, re-arrange and update as appropriate.
- Search the Internet for advice and watch different YouTube tutorials. Most institutional websites have these. You can also search and contribute to Wikipedia or individuals' wikis.

Ethical issues

Ensure your data is protected. When you present your research report, emphasise that you kept your data in a secure locked place such as a safe or on a password-protected computer. Ethics committees are sensitive about these things and may request to see your original documentation about how you ensured ethical conduct throughout your research.

Produce letters to and from participants seeking and granting permission for you to gather and use the data you have collected. Remember that participants have the right to withdraw from the research, and if they do you must destroy all data that refers to them. Keep a record of how participants responded throughout your enquiry. Make sure you maintain the anonymity of participants at all times.

Practical issues

Always back up your files regularly and at least on a daily basis. Keep your data archive active and rearrange entries as different issues emerge. Make sure no one else has access to your data archive without your express permission.

We now turn to the practical issue of how you make sense of this wonderful collection of data and begin to sort and analyse it so that you can generate evidence. This is explained in Chapter 7.

SUMMARY

This chapter has dealt with matters of monitoring practices and gathering data about them. The practices in question are identified as your learning, your actions, other people's learning and other people's actions. All are in transformational mutually reciprocal relationships of influence. You are advised to look for data in all contexts, and suggestions are offered about where to look for the data and how to gather them. Further advice is offered about how to manage the data, with alerts about some potential ethical and practical implications.

Reflective questions

- Can you explain the relationships between your learning and your actions, and between your learning and other people's actions? Why is it important to appreciate these relationships?
- What factors would influence your choice of data-gathering methods?
- Which kind of data do you think might be the most important for your action enquiry?
- When will you gather your data? Will you encounter any difficulties in gathering it?
- How will you manage and store your data? What form will your data archive take?

SEVEN

Turning the data into evidence: testing the validity of claims to knowledge

You now have considerable amounts of data so new questions arise: How do you make sense of it all? How do you present your data so that other people will see what you are getting at? How do you use your data?

This is where you go back to basics.

Remember that the aim of doing research is to create knowledge and theory. A theory is an explanation, often for a practice, and offers reasons and purposes for it. A theory of nursing contains the reasons and purposes of nursing. When you study your practice you learn more about what you are doing; you come to a point where you know something now that you did not know before. This implies also that you can explain what you are doing: you can offer reasons and purposes for your changing practices.

However, when you say, 'I know this', you cannot expect people to believe you unless you produce some kind of evidence to show that what you are saying is true and that they should believe you. This is where you use your data: the data become evidence that you use to ground your knowledge claim. You test the validity of your knowledge claim through scrutinising the evidence and the processes you have used to produce it.

This chapter is organised to show the processes involved in turning the data into evidence and testing the validity of emergent knowledge claims. It contains the following sections:

1. Making claims to knowledge.
2. Identifying criteria and standards of judgement.
3. Selecting data and generating evidence.
4. Procedures for testing the validity of knowledge claims.

1. MAKING CLAIMS TO KNOWLEDGE

When making a claim to knowledge, your first job is to state what the claim is. A reminder: the meaning of 'a knowledge claim' is when you say you know something. You state it both explicitly, as when you say things like, 'I know what I am doing', and implicitly when you say things like, 'Today is Friday', by which you mean, '[I know that] Today is Friday'.

Doing research of any kind is about creating knowledge and generating theory. Doing action research is about this, and it is also about learning to improve practices. The two come together so that action research is understood as being about creating knowledge and generating theory about the processes of improving practices. When you do your action research you can say, '[I am claiming that] [I know that] I have contributed to patients' wellbeing and I can theorise [explain] what I know and how I have come to know it'. You are putting this claim into the public domain for the first time and contributing to the public knowledge base. The knowledge may be about a substantive area such as a clinical aspect or issue of practice, and it can also be about the process of doing research and creating knowledge. Knowledge generated through doing action research is always about both practice and theory. You offer descriptions of what you have done and explanations for why you have done it and what you hope to achieve. Together, these become your personal theories of practice.

Communicating your knowledge

We now introduce a new idea, about what is involved in communicating your knowledge. We explore the idea that there are different levels of communication that move from description to explanation to explication.

Recall the idea set out in Chapter 2 that there are different kinds of knowledge, and that each builds on and develops the other. A basic kind of knowledge is 'know-that', knowledge about facts and artefacts (see Chapter 1). To test the validity of your claim that you know that certain things exist or are the case, you often back up your knowledge claims with empirical data: you point to objects that are or represent real-world artefacts. When you work with 'know-that' forms, you offer mainly descriptions of practice. For example:

> Joe is a student nurse who is learning how to apply wound dressings. As part of his training, he goes to the dressings room with his mentor and considers the different kinds of dressings stacked neatly on shelves, according to their different functions. His mentor asks him, 'Which dressing will you choose for

Mr Grey's leg wound?' Joe chooses a dressing. He says to his mentor, 'I know which dressing to use'. This constitutes knowledge of wound dressings: it stays at the level of what Boyer (1990) called 'knowledge discovery' and does not yet move into the level of theorising. Joe knows about dressings; he knows that one kind is more appropriate than another, but he has not yet articulated how he intends to use the dressing in practice. His claim to 'know-that' is valid but still limited to the level of 'know about a topic'.

In nursing (or any other practice) it is not enough only to have information about something; you also need to be able to integrate knowing about the thing and knowing how to use it, what Ryle (1949) called 'know-how'. Boyer (1990) called this 'a scholarship of integration', the integration of know-that with know-how. You back up your claims by demonstrating how you do things. Know-how is linked with skills and competences.

Joe's mentor asks him, 'How do you use this particular dressing?' Joe is able to show his mentor how the dressing works, and how he intends to use it. His claim that 'I know how to use this dressing' is therefore valid. He can integrate 'know-that' with 'know-how'.

A more refined level of understanding, and therefore achieving a higher level of explanatory adequacy, is when his mentor asks Joe why he chooses this dressing rather than another. In this case Joe can say how he applies his knowledge in the practice setting. Through doing this he demonstrates what Boyer (1990) called 'a scholarship of application'. Evidence for this kind of knowledge can be seen when know-that and know-how are integrated with a new layer of 'know-why'. Joe says: 'I can explain to you why I have chosen this particular dressing and why it is the most appropriate kind. I can also show you how to apply the dressing and explain why I do it this way'. Now he integrates know-that, know-how and know-why.

However, it has to be recognised that much professional knowledge works at and is embedded in a tacit level. Polanyi (1958) speaks about personal knowledge, that is, when we say 'I know' but cannot necessarily explain what we are doing. He says that we know more than we can say. To try this out, ask someone to explain how windscreen wipers work and watch what happens. Personal knowledge involves personal forms of knowing, often embodied, often intuitive or learned from experience. Benner (1984) also spoke about how tacit knowledge emerges over time and through practice into explicit knowledge. Evidence of this kind of knowledge is in the practice, which then transforms into praxis, that is, wise, committed and intentional action. Knowledge of practice needs to be communicated in practical terms through showing its use value in the personal and social world. In a nursing context you would demonstrate praxis when you care for a person through integrating all your capacities of know-that, know-how and know-why as knowledge-of-practice. Schön (1995) calls this 'knowing-in-practice'. When you do this you demonstrate a high level of nursing expertise: you know how and why you practise as you do, and you can explain this to other people.

This kind of knowledge of practice is the basis of the generation of theory. You can say that you have generated your personal theory of practice through explaining what you do at these different levels: this also means that you move from explanation to explication, that is, you can say how and why you make your explanations explicit. When you explain something it is not enough to say that you are claiming to know at different levels; you also have to make explicit the process of how and why you came to know. You have to explain this to your listener or reader. You move from *saying* what you have done to *communicating* what you have done and articulating its significance; you move from telling the story to thinking about how you are communicating the story (see Bereiter and Scardamalia's (1987) idea of moving from knowledge telling to knowledge transforming). This capacity for communicating your knowledge now moves you into the field of generating theory, when you can articulate what you know, how you have come to know it, why you needed to know it, and why your knowledge is important. You also need to say who your knowledge is important for and why it is important. If you can do this you can say that you have generated your personal theory of practice and communicate its significance for your own and other people's learning. (These ideas are explained in greater detail in McNiff, 2014, 2015, 2016.)

Knowledge claims work at all levels. At whatever level you choose to work, you can make knowledge claims: know-that, know-how, personal knowing, capacity to explain and capacity to communicate. You could say:

- I know that certain kinds of wounds require a particular kind of dressing. I know the differences between different kinds of wounds and dressings.
- I know how to identify different kinds of wound and select appropriate kinds of dressings and I know how to apply them.
- I know how to integrate my knowledge of dressings and wounds and why it is important to know it.
- I know the importance of sensitivity when applying dressings to deep wounds. I have learned this from my own experience of injuring my leg and also from applying dressings to patients' wounds.
- I can explain all this to my professional mentor, and by doing so I can claim that I have raised my level of explanatory capacity and therefore my level of professionalism.

You would gather data about all these aspects of your knowledge of practice. The job now is to extract evidence from the data you collect. The first step in this task is to identify criteria and standards of judgement.

2. IDENTIFYING CRITERIA AND STANDARDS OF JUDGEMENT

Making a judgement about the success or quality of anything involves setting criteria and standards of judgement. Criteria are those things you set in advance, and take the form of expectations. If you go to a hotel, you expect the hotel to be clean, warm and welcoming. Cleanliness, warmth and welcome become criteria. When you look at hotels on the Internet you choose which hotel you go to in term of its published criteria. Standards are different though related. If you had to choose between two hotels you would ask, 'How clean? How welcoming?' and you would look on hotel websites at users' reviews to help you decide. Standards are when you make a value judgement about something; you expect the thing to come up to standard.

In nursing practices you can have different criteria and standards of all kinds, and these often work according to different people's interests and values. For example, in the UK many professional practices are judged in terms of whether or not practitioners achieve specified targets. Ambulances are expected to get to an emergency scene within a stipulated time, and the effectiveness of accident and emergency units is judged in terms of how quickly patients are treated. These kinds of criteria tend to work in the interests of the organisation rather than of patients (see Chapter 2). When you make judgements about your own practice it is not enough to say, 'I know which wound dressing to apply and I know how to do it'. You also have to explain the nature of what you did and why you think its quality is good.

It is also not enough to show that you have achieved nominated criteria on assessment documents, though this is important (and is what some organisations require people to do, a kind of tick-box system). You also have to make a judgement about how well you performed the action, which involves your explaining which standards you use. This is especially important in contemporary times of scandals in healthcare and of a number of enquiries into serious shortcomings in care standards by nurses (as reported in Francis, 2013). To show the importance of appropriate professional standards, consider the following.

In a Parliamentary debate, Lord Mancroft told the House of Lords about his experience in the Royal United Hospital, Bath, as follows:

The nurses who looked after me – not all of them; we should never generalise and there were one or two wonderful ones – were mostly grubby, with dirty fingernails and hair. They were slipshod, lazy and, worst of all, drunken and promiscuous. How do I know that? If you are a patient, lying in a bed and being nursed from either side, the nurses talk across you as if you are not there. I know exactly what they got up to the night before. I know how much they drank and what they were planning to do the next night, and it was pretty horrifying. (Hansard, 2008)

At the time, this comment by Lord Mancroft was attacked by nursing associations and other politicians, but it seemed to contribute to changing the climate to one where nurses could be criticised directly for poor standards. It also signalled a change in the discourses whereby politicians could no longer simply refer to nurses as 'angels' and hope to garner personal support. Similarly, the sad and harrowing description by Ann Clwyd, a Labour Member of Parliament, of the poor standards of care related to her husband's death criticised the role of nurses in delivering poor quality care (*The Telegraph*, 2012). The comment from *The Telegraph* was significant:

> There are many excellent nurses in the NHS but it has long been apparent that poor nursing is not some isolated incident but is widespread in many hospitals. Something fundamental has gone wrong with the way nurses are trained and managed. Yet to say as much has, until now, invited the charge of being hostile to the health service. This heartfelt intervention by a prominent Labour politician [Ann Clwyd] may finally encourage a more realistic debate on the subject. It is significant that Jeremy Hunt chose to address the issue head-on recently in his first major speech as Health Secretary. Accepting that there is a problem has taken far too long. For the sake of the NHS, solutions must be found more speedily. (*The Telegraph*, 2012)

Comments such as these corroborate the fact that there is a good deal of systemic/anecdotal evidence of an apparent lack of empathy and compassion in many contemporary nursing practices.

Yet this issue of the need to improve the quality of nursing practices returns us to the central theme of this book, which is that the dominant form of epistemology appears to be the basis of the problem (recall that 'epistemology' involves a theory of knowledge and a theory of knowledge acquisition and creation). The dominant form of knowledge and the way of thinking (logic) remains propositional and technical; these underpinning commitments at a conceptual level transform into the same kinds of commitments at a real-world practical level. The technical-rational epistemological culture remains firmly lodged in people's minds and emerges as technical rational practices for a technical-rational culture. This interview data with a former student nurse shows this in action.

During my clinically based experience I called in a senior nurse because I was concerned about the worsening condition of the patient. The senior nurse came in, checked the patient's monitors, looked at the infusion set and said, 'What's the problem?'. I carefully moved back the blankets to show him that the patient was actually bleeding quite profusely from his post-op wound. The senior nurse than took the lead in dealing with the situation. When discussing this later, he said he was quite shocked at the realisation that he had checked the monitors before the patient. He said, 'Maybe I need to go back to basics'.

The problem continues. It remains the case that senior leadership in nursing often sound somewhat self-congratulatory as they speak about the more technocratic aspects of the extended role of the professional nurse (see Royal College of Nursing, 2005, 2012). Significantly, many current senior nurse leaders qualified at a time when academic and technical knowledge and standards had already become valued more than interpersonal experiential knowledge and standards; the focus on technical rational knowledge continues to be regarded by many senior nurses as a great leap forward. Sadly it has also led nursing away from an 'other-centred' identity as a profession of 'caring doers' to a new self-centred identity as a professional body who can confidently take their places alongside doctors and other professionals.

This has implications for you. As a practising nurse, you are legally responsible for your own professional practice. It is no good saying, 'I was following orders'. You are legally responsible. Consequently, as well as demonstrating respect for organisational targets, you should also set your own standards of practice and judgement, in negotiation with others, and explain how you are fulfilling them: and you are entitled to do so. The kinds of standards of practice and judgement for NHS staff and clinicians are set out clearly in the Berwick Report:

1. Participate actively in the improvement of systems of care.
2. Acquire the skills to do so.
3. Speak up when things go wrong.
4. Involve patients as active partners and co-producers in their own care. (2013: 38)

And:

- Place the quality and safety of patient care above all other aims for the NHS. (This, by the way, is your safest and best route to lower cost.)
- Engage, empower, and hear patients and carers throughout the entire system, and at all times.
- Foster wholeheartedly the growth and development of all staff, especially with regard to their ability and opportunity to improve the processes within which they work.
- Insist upon, and model in your own work, thorough and unequivocal transparency, in the service of accountability, trust, and the growth of knowledge. (2013: 44–45)

This means you need to be able to describe, explain and explicate your practices; you need to know facts and skills and how to integrate them, and you also need to be able to communicate the processes involved. You need to ask yourself whether you live out your own values of care, compassion, competence, communication, courage and commitment, and show how these values come to stand as your professional standards.

You also need to be able to communicate these ideas to others, so that they can see how you make wise judgements about what you are doing. This all means being able to theorise your practice. Further, if you are on a formal course of study at a university, you also need to show how you fulfil the criteria and standards for judging the quality of your academic work as well as your practices, and to what standard (see Chapter 8). This means you are able to integrate practical knowledge with academic knowledge. You show the legitimacy of your practice as a valid form of theory generation, and you show yourself as a competent theorist as well as a capable practitioner.

3. SELECTING DATA AND GENERATING EVIDENCE

Now consider the processes involved in generating evidence that you can use as the basis of testing the validity of your knowledge claims. 'Validity' means, broadly speaking, 'truthfulness': the aim is to show people that they can believe you. Consequently, it is not only the validity of the knowledge claim that is on trial, but of you, the researcher. You show your honour and integrity by showing respect for methodological rigour and for appropriate standards in research.

Multiple aspects are involved in these issues. Two of the most important are:

- analysing and interpreting data;
- generating evidence.

Analysing and interpreting data

When you analyse your data you look for specific things. First you look for the existence of specific pieces of data that you will drag out of your data archive and drop into your evidence archive (see below). To make decisions about which pieces of data you will select as evidence, you first need to analyse your data. Here are some guidelines about how you might do this.

Analysing data

- Compile a data archive containing all your data, sorted into categories (Chapter 6).
- Read your data carefully and become thoroughly familiar with what the data are saying. Sometimes you can be taken by surprise by the data, such as when people say things you did not expect them to say.
- Identify themes that are important to your study: for example, patients' responses to treatments, colleagues' comments on innovative strategies. This becomes a coding exercise, or thematic analysis, which involves categorising your data according to identified themes and concepts.
- Draw up some kind of categorisation system indicating which data go where, and showing when and where the data were gathered.

Interpreting data

You interpret your data according to what you are looking for, that is, your identified criteria. It is important to bring a critical stance to this work because you need to check that you are actually reading what the data say, not what you wish the data would say. For example, following a practice session a senior nurse may say to a junior nurse, 'You did your best'. On the surface this could sound positive, though it may have negative connotations too.

A major issue in interpreting data is when you find data that tell you what you do not want to hear. This is called 'disconfirming data'. You have various options: you can sweep it under the carpet and pretend that the data and the issue it refers to do not exist. This is a common escape route used by many researchers, but is not the most helpful or educational. Much better is to face up to the situation that the data are showing and use them as a useful steer to show you that you are on the wrong track and need to get back onto the right one.

Analysing and interpreting data are key precursors to generating evidence.

Generating evidence

Evidence is not the same as data. Data are all those pieces of information you gather throughout your enquiry to show what is happening. Evidence relates to those specific pieces of data that show criteria in action. We have said throughout this book that you judge your practices in terms of your values. Can you show that you are demonstrating care and compassion? Can you produce feedback from others to show that you are not simply saying this but that it really is the case?

There is a reasonably straightforward procedure for generating evidence from your data, as follows (see Figure 7.1):

1. Identify criteria for judging whatever issue you wish to judge. If it is about your practice you will probably judge the quality of practice in terms of whether you live your values in your practice. Your values become your criteria. Examples of criteria are:

   - Care: do you demonstrate kindness to patients?
   - Compassion: do you listen to patients?
   - Efficiency: do you use the right procedures at the right time?

   Similarly, if the issue concerns your research you will probably judge the quality of your research in the same terms. For example:

   - Discipline: do you demonstrate methodological rigour?
   - Honesty: do you show that you have read the literatures you are citing and not just name-dropping?
   - Independent enquiry: do you test out your own ideas and are you prepared to engage with issues in the literatures?

2. Search your database and select those pieces of data that show your values in action. For example, you could select an email from your mentor congratulating you on your efficiency in helping a patient; or you could produce extracts from a tape-recorded conversation where you are discussing the best way to help a diabetic remain stable.

3. Drag those pieces of data out of your data archive and drop them into a new evidence archive, just as you do when you drag and drop something on your computer, or transfer something from one bag to another. Inevitably the pieces of evidence you generate will be fewer than your pieces of data because some of your data may not show you what you are looking for. Tape-recorded conversations will probably include pleasantries or comments about the weather, which would not stand as evidence that would ground your knowledge claims, so you would discard those data as irrelevant.

4. Aim to take your complete data archive with you if you are going to an examination, especially for academic accreditation. Your examiners are entitled to ask to see your evidence so it would be embarrassing not to have it to hand, let alone jeopardise the credibility of your practice and research.

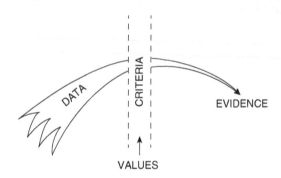

Figure 7.1 Transforming data into evidence

Important points to watch out for

Important points to watch out for when generating evidence include:

- gathering multiple sources of evidence;
- ensuring the authenticity of the evidence;
- triangulation;
- developing an evidence trail for all aspects of your research. (See also Yin, 2009: 114–124)

Gathering multiple sources of evidence

Aim to gather multiple sources of evidence. It is not enough only to have evidence from tape-recorded interviews or from personal journals. This would show lack of responsibility in producing a broad enough base from which to make knowledge claims. In an action enquiry you could draw evidence from any or all of the following: personal logs, audio or videotape-recorded interactions and interviews, surveys and participants' feedback. You could probably draw on many other sources, depending on the research question and aim. You would probably also produce documentary evidence from public documents and policy statements.

Ensuring the authenticity of the evidence

The pieces of evidence you produce need to show their authenticity. Any reports submitted as evidence need to indicate the source, including information about who generated the report and its date and location. Photographs should be dated and, if possible, signed by the persons in the photos to show their authenticity and agreement to have the photo used. Responses from patients should ideally have the patient's signature and be dated. It is easy to fudge data and pretend that things happened when they didn't, and famous cases are cited about how researchers actually fabricated their data. It is possible sometimes to get away with such practices but there is always the likelihood that falsity will be revealed, so stay true to your values and produce a fine evidence base that you can be proud of.

Triangulation

This is a common procedure for testing the validity of evidence, where you generate evidence through examination of at least two data sources that focus on the same point, and ideally more than two. For example, if you wished to show the effectiveness of a new procedure you could look at the following: record sheets to show what had been done; feedback from patient questionnaires to show their responses to the procedure; your reflective journal to show your views and experiences; comments from colleagues' texts about their experiences; and many other sources. Also, triangulation can happen in different ways. Williamson et al. cite Denzin (1989) as identifying:

- data triangulation, involving many different data collection sources;
- investigator triangulation, involving more than one researcher to collect and analyse data;
- theoretical triangulation, involving more than one theoretical approach (for example, Marxist, feminist and/or phenomenological perspectives) to interpret findings;
- methodological triangulation, of which there are two types. 'Within method' triangulation involves using different data collection methods within one paradigm. 'Between method' triangulation involves the use of qualitative and quantitative data collection approaches within one study to investigate the same phenomenon. (Williamson et al., 2012: 34)

You could choose whichever triangulation methods were appropriate for the level of sophistication of your study, but you definitely do need to show that you have triangulated your data in some way, otherwise the research would be weakened methodologically.

Developing an evidence trail for all aspects of your research

Aim to generate evidence for all aspects of your research. For example, when you ask: 'What issue do I wish to investigate? What is my concern?' you would produce data and generate evidence that showed your concern in action. As a hospital manager you would produce statistical evidence to show that too many nurses are leaving their jobs; as a ward sister you would produce documentary evidence to show that patients were happy with the quality of care. You would produce evidence for each question in your research story. On page 106 we outlined some of the forms of data you could look for: the aim now is to turn some of those data into evidence.

NB: some researchers have critiqued the idea of aiming for commensurability of opinion through triangulation. Laws, for example, points out that:

> Accounts collected from different perspectives may not match tidily at all. There may be mismatch and even conflict between them. A mismatch does not necessarily mean that the data collection is flawed – it could be that people just have very different accounts of similar phenomena. (Laws, 2003: 281, cited in Bell, 2005: 116)

Mason also points out:

> The idea [of triangulation] is that, if you measure the same phenomenon from different angles or positions, you will get an accurate reading or measurement of it. This is problematic because ... different methods and data sources are likely to throw light onto different social or ontological phenomena or research questions. ... Furthermore, it implies a view of the social world which says that there is one, objective, and knowable social reality, and all that social researchers have to do, is to work out which are the most appropriate triangulation points to measure it by – a view with which many researchers in the qualitative tradition would of course take issue. (2002: 190)

We agree. It is not possible to legislate meanings with which everyone will agree. If we claim to live in pluralistic societies we need to live our values in relation to data gathering, analysis and interpretation too, recognising that different people and cultures live by different values and therefore have different criteria and standards. This point can lead to deep philosophical debates about whether there are universal values. Who says that cruelty to children is wrong? How do they justify this stance? What is cruelty? What is a child? These are difficult questions that often lead to situations of intractable conflict.

4. PROCEDURES FOR TESTING THE VALIDITY OF KNOWLEDGE CLAIMS

Now consider the procedures involved when testing the validity of knowledge claims as potential public knowledge, that is, they are judged as appropriate for placing in the public domain.

When you make a claim to knowledge you are implicitly saying that it is a valid claim. Validity, as noted, means that people can believe you. It indicates your trustworthiness as a researcher and a practitioner. However, if you make a claim such as 'I am carrying out this procedure better than before', you cannot expect other people to believe you unless you (a) produce authenticated evidence to support and ground your claim and (b) check with other people that they feel you are justified in making the claim. You may like to think that you are justified in claiming something but other people may have different opinions. You can check that you are justified in claiming it through first demonstrating that you have interrogated your data, taken steps to authenticate the evidence, and generated evidence according to the kinds of validity checks outlined above. This counts towards the process of establishing personal validity. Now you need to check that other people agree with your opinion, which counts towards establishing social validity. You can do this by using different forms of validation.

Forms of validation

There are many different forms of validation but two of the most useful for your project are personal, or self-validation, and social validation.

Personal validation or self-validation

This is where you check your findings against your own criteria in the form of your values. When you look at your evidence in relation to the values you have identified as criteria, do you see those values in action? However, this is where things become problematic and interesting.

Technically you would draw out of your evidence base those pieces that show your values in action and that contribute to the validity of your knowledge claim. Say participation was a core value for you, and you wanted to get more participation from others in finding new ways to care for people with dementia.

You may decide to interview colleagues about practices, and you may also decide to interview patients with dementia themselves, to find out what their experiences are. However, this may get you into trouble in several ways: you may incur the wrath of ethics committees who forbid the involvement of vulnerable people in the research (in this case, patients with dementia); you may find that not all your colleagues agree with your value of universal participation; you may also find that your idea of participation does not match other people's ideas about participation. Some may hold a one-sided view that 'participation' means that they ask questions that others answer, whereas you hold a view that everyone is entitled to ask questions so all are involved. Therefore, saying that you have tested the validity of your evidence by showing how you are living your values in your practices can be problematic, given that we live in pluralistic societies where everyone has a different opinion about what is right and defensible. Facing up to dilemmas like this means that you need to negotiate the steps involved in your action enquiry at all times with all participants, and keep records of what you are doing. If ever you are challenged, you have your records to show that you respected all protocols and did everything you could to ensure correct ethical practice.

At all times aim to check out with all participants that they are comfortable with the approach you have developed about your research. Check especially that you are not breaching ethical guidelines or stepping on toes anywhere. This can be time consuming but is worthwhile in terms of enhanced relationships and permission to proceed with your research. This then turns into a process of social validation.

Social validation

This is where others test the validity of your knowledge claims in light of your evidence and your interpretation of its meaning and significance. People involved in exercises to establish validity can include:

Peers: You invite your colleagues to scrutinise your evidence base, show them how you have arrived at your provisional knowledge claims and invite their critical responses. Your peers could include colleagues, patients, patients' families, managers, academic supervisors and study group participants, and any other persons who have a stake in or are interested in your project.

Academic validation: If you are on an award-bearing course you would need to demonstrate methodological rigour through carrying out meticulous validation procedures. You would also need to explain what you have done to show that you are able to engage in scholarly debate, and you would need to explain that you have observed academic criteria and achieved appropriate academic standards.

Setting up a validation group: When you present your work to a group of peers, whether in a clinical practice or formal academic setting, you would need to convene a validation group. The job of the group is to consider your claims, scrutinise your data, and read your reports of how you have generated evidence from the data and why you feel entitled to make a claim to improved practices. Their job is to give you critical feedback about the quality of your work so that you can proceed or go back and review specific elements. Your validation group would comprise individuals whose opinions and capacity for making wise and balanced judgements you trust. Sometimes others, such as your academic tutor or professional mentor will make decisions about who is on the validation panel. This is fine because you need to feel confident that you can show that you have generated high-quality evidence, and that you can explain the processes involved to anyone and defend your position. At any point in a validation meeting you will probably be challenged to explain something. Be prepared to engage with these challenges, and show your knowledge by explaining how you have studied and improved your practices, and, where appropriate, make sure you can relate what you have done to key issues in the literatures.

SUMMARY

This chapter has outlined how to turn data into evidence. It has revisited the idea of making claims to knowledge, generating evidence from the data, and testing the validity of the evidence and the claims. Ideas regarding matters of criteria and standards of judgement are offered, as well as information on how to analyse and interpret data for generating evidence. Advice is given regarding procedures for testing the validity of knowledge claims, and for validation procedures.

Reflective questions

- Are you confident about what making a knowledge claim means and involves?
- Do you appreciate how different levels of knowledge claim comprise different levels and forms of knowledge?
- What procedures are involved in analysing and interpreting data? How do you generate evidence from the data?
- What kinds of criteria would you identify for your action enquiry?
- Will you be able to develop appropriate procedures for testing the validity of your own knowledge claims? What do you think they will be and how will you arrange for them?

III

SIGNIFICANCE OF YOUR ACTION RESEARCH

This part is about making your research public, and demonstrating its significance for different contexts and dimensions.

It contains Chapter 8 and 9.

CHAPTER 8   WRITING UP YOUR ACTION RESEARCH

This chapter outlines what is involved in writing up your action research. It explains the difference between validity and legitimacy, and emphasises the importance of establishing the legitimacy of your action research for different contexts and dimensions. Different forms of texts are described as well as the different audiences for whom they may be written. Advice is offered about developing good writing skills and habits. The need to make your work public becomes a special issue, for this is where you can find ways of influencing new directions for nursing and nursing research.

CHAPTER 9   THE SIGNIFICANCE OF YOUR ACTION RESEARCH

This chapter discusses the importance of communicating the significance of your action research for different groupings and dimensions, including the personal, the professional and the political. In the personal dimension the main aspects of significance are that you show how you demonstrate that you are a capable practitioner and theorist. The professional dimension is that you are able to exercise your educational influence in the thinking of others, including those in your own organisation.

The political significance is that you are able to contribute to public debates about who should own nursing knowledge, and the need for the development of nursing as a broad-based profession that includes and recognises all those involved in caring for patients.

This part gives advice on disseminating your research findings most effectively. It explains the significance of doing so for nursing and the nursing profession. It encourages you to make your contribution to the knowledge base and values base of nursing for the good of the most important group – the patients.

EIGHT

Writing up your action research

This chapter is about writing up your action research. Writing up is an essential part of doing research, because it demonstrates that you have carried out a high quality piece of work whose value and importance should be recognised by others. You also show that doing research qualifies you to speak for yourself and have your ideas taken seriously. You are not speaking out of opinion or ignorance, but from an informed evidence-based position. Others have tested the validity of your knowledge claims and agreed that what you say is trustworthy. This is especially important for clinical nurses, because it positions them as legitimately in charge of their practices, and able to make contributions to public debates about what counts as nursing, who owns nursing knowledge and how decisions about quality should be made. Effectively, writing up your research for public dissemination and critique enables you to contribute to reclaiming nursing as a patient-centred profession.

This chapter outlines some of these issues and contains the following points:

1. The importance of demonstrating validity and legitimacy.
2. Writing and the production of texts: possible structures, different kinds of reports, how to write them, who writes them.
3. Developing writing skills and capacities: developing habits and routines; nuts and bolts of good writing practices.
4. Making your work public: conferences, papers, books, articles, social media.
5. Contributing to the public knowledge base.

1. THE IMPORTANCE OF DEMONSTRATING VALIDITY AND LEGITIMACY

There is a difference between the ideas of validity and legitimacy, and both are important for showing that you and your work are to be taken seriously. Here is a story to show the difference.

> Some years ago, as charge nurse on a medical paediatric ward, I encountered a dilemma that highlights for me the difference between validity and legitimacy. We had a child admitted who, in addition to the primary reason for admission, also had some minor injuries, including bruising. A protocol was in place for dealing with these situations, which of course we followed. The parents appeared to be a caring couple and were easily able to explain the injuries. All this was noted, recorded and communicated through the correct channels. A complication arose when a care assistant who worked on the ward approached me to say that a friend had recently picked her up after work, seen the parents leaving and commented that they were neighbours of hers, and that on a couple of occasions when passing their house she had heard a child screaming, to the extent that she wondered if she should notify the police or other authorities. I thanked the nursing assistant for raising this and discussed it confidentially with other senior staff. There was a deep division between those who felt that this changed the way we perceived the relationship between the parents and child, and those who angrily felt that this was no more than gossip. My own view was that any information that could protect a child was valid and we had a responsibility to take it into account. The problem for some people was that they felt this was not a legitimate way of collecting information.

Experiences like this happen every day. Clinical nurses are caught in dilemmas about being able to demonstrate the validity of what they are saying within a social or political context that often denies them legitimacy. As noted throughout, the legitimacy of nurses to say what counts as professional practices remains open to challenge. The challenges are strengthened because the main vehicle for the legitimation of nursing knowledge is through publication, but a glance at most journals shows that the majority of articles do not come from nurses working in clinical areas. It is still accepted that academic nurses have the right kind of nursing knowledge that qualifies them to write for publication. This view that only academic nurses are able to say what counts as nursing and who is able to do it (themselves) has taken nursing away from the patient and into the university. By writing for publication, clinical nurses can change this situation.

Yet this is where clinical nurses themselves often become their own worst enemies. Because we are all born into a culture with its established habitus, we learn not to question what the culture tells us. A certain stasis tends to set in and the wheel of power continues: systems protect and perpetuate themselves through specific strategies of power, including the spreading of misinformation. Nurses come to believe the misinformation they are told, in this case, that they are not able to write, especially for publication.

However, they can easily break into and open up this closed situation to public scrutiny. This does take work, but the work has the potential for cultural change. A main way to do it is through deciding to develop your capacity for writing.

2. WRITING AND THE PRODUCTION OF TEXTS

This section is about how you can write and produce different kinds of texts for different audiences, and why you need to do so.

As a clinical nurse you could write at least two kinds of texts for dissemination. The first would be a work-based report for a peer professional audience, the second for an academic audience if you are on a formal university degree course. Both kinds of report could also be written up for journal publication.

First, look at how you write a work-based report.

Writing a work-based report for a peer professional audience

Whether you are writing for your workplace peers or for an academic audience, aim to write a report that communicates the process of doing your action research. It involves asking questions like these (as outlined on page 21):

- What do I want to investigate?
- Why do I want to investigate it?
- How do I monitor practices and gather data to show what the situation is like?
- What methodology and methods will I use?
- What actions will I take to try to achieve my overall aims?
- How will I continue to gather data and generate evidence to show that what I am saying is well grounded?
- How will I test the validity of my provisional conclusions?
- How will I explain the significance of my research?
- How will I do things differently in future? How will I modify my thinking and actions in light of my evaluation?

When you come to write up the story, at a basic level you turn these planning questions, which you write in the future tense, into a story that you tell in the past tense, as follows:

- What did I want to investigate?
  You set the context and state the research issue and research question.

- Why did I want to investigate it?
  You explain why this was an issue worthy of investigation and describe some relevant contexts.

- How did I show what the situation was like?
  You explain how you monitored practices and gathered data to show what the situation and its contexts were like.

- What methodology and methods did I use?
  You explain which methodology you used, including how you planned and designed your research, gathered data, identified participants, ensured ethical conduct and considered other practical issues (remember that methodology is different from methods).

- What actions did I take to try to achieve my overall aims?
  You outline the practical actions you took.

- How did I continue to gather data and generate evidence to show that what I was saying was well grounded?
  You explain how you continued monitoring practice and gathering data and now began to generate evidence. Explain how this involved data analysis and interpretation.

- How did I test the validity of my provisional conclusions?
  Explain how you tested the validity of your findings drawing on other people's feedback.

- How do I explain the significance of my research?
  Say how you feel you are contributing to other people's thinking as well as continuing to develop your own. Say that you are hoping to contribute to new thinking about your profession.

- How am I doing things differently? How have I modified my thinking and actions in light of my evaluation?
  Say how you are thinking and doing things differently because you engaged in your action enquiry.

Here is a story to show how you can do this.

Taking action in a psychiatric setting

What did I want to investigate?

Here you set the context and state the research issue and research question.

> I am a nurse manager of a small psychiatric unit made up of three wards, each of 15 beds, admitting patients from different geographical areas. Some of our patients come with acute psychiatric conditions for the first time. Others are long-term community-based people with recurring psychiatric issues. This story is about a six-month project colleagues and I undertook in our unit.

We like to think we developed a new dynamic culture that contributed to patients' enhanced sense of wellbeing.

At the time I was a newly appointed clinical nurse manager, and I was not comfortable with the existing culture of the unit. The running of the wards was based on the assumption that people would be admitted for a few days, be treated and supported with their condition, and then discharged. However, the reality was that, whether for social or community reasons or the failure to respond to treatment, people were frequently with us for longer periods than originally anticipated. This often led to some patients' developing a feeling that they were leading a directionless existence, which was manifestly demotivating for the people themselves and for the staff supporting them. Despite inputs from other departments such as occupational therapy, which people could attend on a voluntary basis, it was common to see patients sitting listlessly around the clinical area and not engaged in any meaningful or productive activity. This went against my personal and professional values that all people should enjoy life as much as possible and, from a clinical perspective, realise as fully as possible their potential for engaging in a productive and rewarding life.

I decided to set up an informal collaborative research project with colleagues to investigate how we could transform the current situation into a productive and life-affirming experience where people would feel inspired to engage and try to realise their potential for maximum wellbeing, depending on their circumstances. We set ourselves a research question: How do we encourage greater engagement by patients in realising their potential for maximum wellbeing, depending on their circumstances? Two of our colleagues were registered for Masters programmes, so they took the opportunity to write the project up from their separate perspectives. This was useful for us all because it introduced us also to works in the literature by, for example, Fromm (1956) who speaks about the need for loving and productive relationships as the basis for a full life, and Frankl (1959) who speaks about the human search for meaning. We also read writings from Seligman (2011) who speaks about the need for happiness and human flourishing, and from Noddings' (1984) work on caring.

Why did I want to investigate this issue?
You explain why this was an issue worthy of investigation and set out some relevant contexts.

Doing this research was important because people who are already prone to recurring bouts of depression or other psychiatric problems spending time unengaged and inactive is demotivating and can have a depressive effect. The experience also tended to have a demotivating effect on other patients who come into the area, and evoked the general impression of a temporary dumping ground for people who were not coping with society. As a staff we understood the needs of some individuals for asylum from the pressures of everyday life, and we understood that the chance to get away and recover in our supported unit could be useful, but we did not feel that sitting around listlessly for long periods of the day was helping.

How did I show what the situation was like?

You explain how you monitored practices and gathered data to show what the situation and its contexts were like.

We decided to conduct an action enquiry, so began by identifying a research issue and explaining why it was an issue. We gathered data informally to provide a baseline that would give us a steer on what was happening and how we might take action. Our data showed that despite the existence of activity plans for most patients, the attendance level was often low and many patients would stay in bed until very late morning. This meant they missed meals and physical activities and were in danger of promoting physical degeneration. A snapshot image when passing through the patient areas showed numbers of people sitting around not engaging or interacting, despite the ready availability of ward-based and occupational therapy activities.

What methodology and methods did I use?

You explain which methodology you used, including how you planned and designed your research, gathered data, identified participants, ensured ethical conduct and considered other practical issues (remember that methodology is different from methods).

We began our action enquiry by articulating the research issue and explaining why it was an issue. We decided that this would be a collaborative research project, involving patients and their families or carers. It had to be collaborative because it focused directly on encouraging the patients to change their own thinking and actions. Based on observation and feedback we identified lack of physical activity as the central feature of the problem, so decided to introduce a programme of exercises. As a common-sense formality the medical team were asked for their agreement about the appropriateness of each individual patient taking part in some gentle activities. As well as the patients, we checked with the families; they were fully in agreement, and we involved them in planning the programme. In the event many joined in when they were visiting and offered help wherever possible. We also drew up a brief proposal for the hospital ethics committee. They automatically approved it on the grounds that what we were planning was a rehabilitation initiative that we would normally undertake.

What actions did I take to try to achieve my overall aims?

You outline the practical actions you took.

Colleagues and I identified the main problem as lack of physical activity. When we raised this at staff meetings or at individual and group meetings with patients, there was general agreement that activity levels were low and that this was not conducive to a healthy lifestyle. So, in discussion with other staff and with patient groups we devised a programme of physical activity and set about introducing it. The programme had to allow for varying age groups and levels of fitness. It was also important to consider how to sustain it in an often unpredictable and usually busy working area where ordinary levels of clinical observation had to be high, and with no spare staff capacity.

We agreed to start with a 30-minute activity session each morning, which would be led by an identified member of staff or a patient, often working together, on a daily basis. We encouraged all patients, and any staff who wished to or were available, to participate according to their level of ability and confidence. On good days this would mean a walk outside for ten minutes followed by some gentle stretches. We kept records of names and numbers attending. This was also recorded in patients' individual notes. Attendance was voluntary but determined attempts were made to persuade people to give it a try. Even if they simply wandered along gently and took small active parts, this would be an increase in their activity levels for many. On some days the weather would not allow going outside so one of the larger indoor spaces would be used. Activities would be changed regularly using basic equipment such as throwing or kicking a ball, or passing a chair around from person to person. Activities lasted for a short period of time and we tried to change them regularly so that they did not become boring or robotic.

As time went on people began to find this more enjoyable than they had expected. We tried to be imaginative and innovative in developing activities. There was a generally humorous and positive response so we extended the idea by introducing a regular evening activity after the last meal. This meant that instead of slumping in front of a television people had the option, and were encouraged, to go outside to throw a ball, look at flowers and birds, or undertake any activity they or staff identified that would be novel and interesting. Different patients or staff would take a lead according to knowledge or expertise. People often commented on how the relationship between many patients and members of staff, and among patients, often became more relaxed, and conversations would arise more spontaneously on more occasions. Our general observation was that self-esteem and social withdrawal issues seemed to be improved by the activity, especially walking programmes.

How did I continue to gather data and generate evidence to show that what I was saying was well grounded?

You explain how you continued monitoring practice and gathering data and now began to generate evidence. Explain how this involved data analysis and interpretation.

> A simple record was kept of names and numbers attending the exercise sessions and a note of activities. The activity was also noted on individual patients' records, and some time was allocated at patients' meetings to discuss existing activities and plan new ones. This was also recorded in the minutes. The simple expedient of recording people's comments about the exercise activities gave an indication as to how positively people felt about them. As this was new activity there was no real baseline to compare it with, but eyeball evidence indicated greater levels of interaction and regular laughter during and after the exercise occasions. The reason for rolling it out into the evening was that a number of patients expressed a wish to do so. This was seen as positive because this is a time of day when many departments have closed down and there is a lull in activities for most patients.

How did I test the validity of my provisional conclusions?

Explain how you tested the validity of your findings drawing on other people's feedback.

> Some positive benefits indicated a change in overall atmosphere. An example of this was when I pointed out to a group of visiting managers that the individual exuberantly swinging from a tree while other people were kicking a ball around was in fact a member of staff who was accompanying the group. Another example was when we had to fill in an accident report about the cut arm of a 76-year-old gentleman who, having been admitted with severe depression, had now sustained his injury whilst diving to take a catch at lawn cricket. We gathered general feedback using informal interviews, and also during patient meetings, therapeutic sessions, discussion with relatives and feedback from staff in other departments. On the whole, everyone felt very positively. Staff could identify benefits in individual patients, visitors liked to see their relatives actively engaged, and other members of staff commented on the general atmosphere and activity levels. Although we did not keep formal records, we saw an increase in the numbers of staff in other areas who expressed an interest in coming to work in our unit. Staff and patients were proud of this level of activity but we did not seek to publicise it in any way outside the groups involved, as this felt somewhat patronising and manipulative of what was for most patients just an enjoyable exercise session. We did not feel we should be seen as capitalising on their conditions.

How do I explain the significance of my research?

Say how you feel you are contributing to other people's thinking as well as continuing to develop your own. Say how you are hoping to contribute to new thinking about your profession.

> The initiative came about through what was effectively reflection-in-action where an issue was noted, followed by further reflection on what we were learning and a consideration of the potential implications. A response was decided upon, tried out and evaluated, and so the cycle continued. With low staffing levels we might easily have accepted that this project was unsustainable, but just by our addressing the issue positively, it achieved some momentum of its own.

> *Mens sana in corpore sano* – this is an ancient concept yet one I feel holds as true today as ever. Endless hours of inactivity do not appear to have any beneficial effect on people at a point when they should be preparing to be more active and return to the community. The findings of our small-scale informal study could have implications for combating tendencies among patients, often intensified by medication, for rising late in the morning.

How am I doing things differently? How have I modified my thinking and actions in light of my evaluation?

Say how you are thinking and doing things differently because you engaged in your action enquiry.

> The benefits of developing a routine of regular activity have become part of our discussions with patients pre-discharge. We also encouraged community support workers to consider implementing a self-generated programme of activities such as a short walk in the morning and some other activity later in the day. We like to think we are influencing new practices in the community. We continue with our modest exercise regimes and hope they help patients recover more quickly and return to everyday living.

Now consider writing a text for academic accreditation.

Writing a text for academic accreditation

If you are on a higher education award-bearing course you can use the same structure as above for your text, whether for a foundation or first degree, a Masters dissertation or a PhD thesis. This would help you achieve the anticipated criteria for all research reports, as follows.

Criteria for all research reports (including action research reports)

All research reports show the achievement of these criteria:

- identify a research issue and articulate a research question;
- demonstrate knowledge of the field and subject matter;
- say why this is an issue, give relevant contexts and link them with the literatures;
- say what has been achieved (reports contain a claim to knowledge);
- describe and explain how it has been achieved;
- explain how ethical matters were respected and catered for;
- provide critical feedback about what the reports are saying (test the validity of the claim so that the story may be believed); and
- outline the significance of the research for new forms of thinking and action. (See McNiff, 2014: 52)

Additional criteria for action research reports

In addition to the above, action research reports contain:

An action story: This is about how you studied a substantive topic or theme, whether from an insider or outsider perspective. You gather data and generate evidence about it. You explain how learning about the topic has enabled you to contribute to improving a particular situation. For example:

- You study diabetes as a topic. You learn about its signs, symptoms and treatments.
- You study the importance of good record keeping.
- You study your work with a patients' group. You maintain a reflective diary about how patients are responding to exercise.

A research story: This is your ongoing explanation for why you did what you did, what you learned through the process, and your articulation of the significance of your action and learning for your own and other people's learning and practices.

Your action story and research story weave into one. They are inseparable, but your reader should see clear elements of action and reflection throughout. They should also see that you are aware of this, through your inclusion of reflective episodes throughout the text.

In action research texts you do these things:

- You tell the story of what you know and how you have come to know it through doing your research.
- You explain how you have tested the validity of your knowledge claims.
- You analyse the significance of the story for your own and other people's learning.

- You explain how you draw on your experience when making judgements about the quality of your actions and research, and how you test it in relation to the experience of others in your current contexts or in the literatures.

Action research texts also do the following:

- They link values and action: Values come to stand as criteria for judging the quality of your action, your research and your text.
- They show sensitivity in ethical matters: You use your judgement for individual cases, and check with seniors in problematic situations. You negotiate permissions with ethics committees as appropriate.
- Stories are told by the 'I', which is implicit throughout: The text is not 'all about me'; the 'me' is of secondary importance. The unit of enquiry is the knowledge claim of the 'I' to have acted educationally and ethically so that others' lives become richer and more fulfilling. Action research is not about making 'interventions', which may often appear as interference. It is about exercising your educational influence in your own and others' thinking so that all can make informed and wise decisions for themselves.

Criteria for action research texts submitted for accreditation

Work submitted for accreditation must also fulfil the following conditions:

- A main criterion at doctoral level is that the thesis makes an original contribution to knowledge of the field: originality is not necessary at Masters or undergraduate level. The field in question is nursing, or a particular area of nursing.
- You demonstrate critical engagement, both with the thinking of other people as communicated through the literatures, and with your own, as you work with your own ideas.
- You demonstrate knowledge of the field (nursing) and appropriate literatures (texts about nursing practices, contexts, knowledge and theory).
- You write about substantive (subject-oriented) and theoretical (theory-oriented) matter.

All texts show the capacity for high-quality communication. This is dealt with now.

3. DEVELOPING WRITING SKILLS AND CAPACITIES

Here are some ideas about how to develop writing habits and routines, and other practicalities of good writing practices.

Developing habits and routines

Many texts about developing your practice as a writer emphasise the need for establishing habits and routines. These include the following.

Practise

No book or person can teach you how to write. You have to learn it for yourself, which means practice. Just as you learn how to swim through swimming, so you also learn to write through writing. Even the most experienced writers had to learn the job through doing the job; there are no short cuts to learning how to write.

Most writers stress the need for hard work. O'Reilly (1984) emphasises that producing a text requires a small amount of talent and a lot of hard work. Tharp writes:

> I will keep stressing the point about creativity being augmented by routine and habit. Get used to it. In these pages [you find] a perennial debate, born in the Romantic era, between the beliefs that all creative acts are born of (a) some transcendent, inexplicable Dionysan act of inspiration, a kiss from God on your brow that allows you to give the world *The Magic Flute*, or (b) hard work.
>
> If it isn't obvious already, I come down on the side of hard work. (2006: 7)

Yes. Don't wait for someone to do it for you. Do it yourself and get on with it.

Habits and routines

Aim to develop good writing habits and routines. These include:

Learn which mode of writing suits you best: Some people write directly onto a computer; others prefer to write longhand and then type onto a computer. Many do a mix and match. Some people produce a draft text on a computer, print it, edit the printed version and re-type. There is no standard format for writing; everyone needs to work out their own way. Aim to try out different strategies and be flexible while you are writing. The main thing is to write and not find excuses not to write.

Begin in the middle: You hear stories of people staring at a blank page waiting for inspiration, which means they will probably wait a long, long time. Don't believe the stories. Writing brings its own inspiration as you write. As you work with ideas and see them take on a life of their own through words and sentences, the ideas begin to flow. You don't need to begin at the beginning. Start anywhere, with any ideas that come to you. Everything, including writing, is always in the middle of something else, and provides its own beginning.

Get on and write: Don't expect things to be perfect first time. Producing a final good quality text requires multiple drafts; this involves editing, revising and rewriting (see below). Don't spend time polishing a first draft because it is all going to change as you refine your text. So don't put it off; just get on and write. The time you spend worrying about what to write could be spent jotting down some keywords, which could lead to fabulous inspiration.

Be prepared to edit, revise and rewrite: Many people work out their ideas through the writing. This means that, by the time you get to the end of a text you wish you could go back and rewrite it, to explore the interesting ideas that have emerged through the writing. Unfortunately this is not often possible if you are working to a deadline, or have to hand in your assignment on time. However, do make time in your schedule for editing, revising and rewriting (see below).

Stay healthy while writing: Aim to stay healthy while writing. Move as much as possible and change your position regularly. You can sit or stand, sit on the bed or armchair, get a kneeling chair – anything to keep your body moving and to stay healthy while physically writing. Drink plenty of water and other fluids to stay hydrated, and keep a small bowl of water on your writing area to maintain humidity (but not near your computer for fear of mishaps). Take short breaks, and learn how much you can write at any one time. For many people this is 20 minutes or one or two hours at a time, but when the ideas begin to flow writing can become compulsive.

Learn which time of day suits you best: Learn which time of day suits you best to write, whether in the morning, evening or in patches throughout the day. No one time is right for everyone. Experiment and find out for yourself. Also use time on buses and in queues to write mentally and physically. Carry a notebook or smartphone for jotting down sentences or for making notes that you will write up later.

Pay attention to family and friends: Don't get so absorbed in your writing that you forget that you have a family and friends who need and love you. Pay attention to them and include them wherever possible. Run ideas past them, and keep them up to date with what you are writing about. They may not fully understand but they will appreciate your trying to involve them.

Keep a record of progress: Keep a record of writing progress, possibly as a diary or log or blog. When you finish writing for the day, make a note of what you are going to write about tomorrow. This lends continuity to your writing, and gives you a flying start to the next day.

Developing good writing practices

Here are some ideas for developing good writing practices.

Write for a reader, not for yourself: This is probably the single most common error that beginning writers make: they assume that their reader knows what they are talking about. Readers don't know; all they know about you and your work is what you tell them, what they read on the page. It is your responsibility to lead your reader through your text. You can do this by inserting sentences that tell them what to look out for. Write alerts such as: 'In this section I speak about …' or 'Here are some ideas from Benner …'. Try to help your reader navigate their way through your text and don't expect them to find their way by themselves. If they get lost they will abandon the reading.

Be prepared to produce multiple drafts: Sometimes people think that their first draft will be the final draft. Sadly it does not work like this. For every final copy that the world sees, multiple drafts are produced, developed and revised. Be prepared for this: do not wait for the right moment to write because it never comes. Just do it.

Spend time on editing, revising and rewriting: Be prepared to spend time on editing, revising and rewriting. Editing happens at different levels in the production of a text. You edit at the level of words, when you take out repetition, find better words and take out frills and padding: 'use' is just as good as 'utilise'. Less is often more in academic and professional texts. Editing also happens at the level of sentences and paragraphs, when you make the text flow easily and meaningfully. This often means inserting sentences that link ideas for continuity.

Many books and Internet resources are available about producing good quality texts. Most higher education institutions post practical and theoretical advice on their websites. Reading these resources will save you a lot of time in the long run.

Now consider how making your work public acts as a means of celebrating your knowledge and making your mark.

4. MAKING YOUR WORK PUBLIC

When you write you make your physical mark on a surface, whether this be on paper or a screen or in the sand. You also make your political mark: you stand up and are counted for what you believe in. Writing therefore becomes the symbolic mark for making your political mark. This means you need to know what to write, how to write it and why you should write it. We have already considered what and how to write: now consider why you should write and what you can achieve through doing so. Key points for attention are:

- your potential audiences;
- form of writing;
- contributing to the knowledge base.

Your potential audiences

Some of your potential audiences are as follows.

People in your workplace

Throughout your project you have talked with workplace colleagues including other nurses, managers, patients and families. Now you need to tell them your findings and say why these are important. You can do this by writing a report and finding ways to disseminate it. First get your line manager's approval and invite their support by requesting a slot at a staff meeting or professional development event. Ask them to write a cover note to endorse the report if they are willing. Aim to communicate your learning through your report and suggest subtly (or not) that colleagues could also study their practices, collaboratively if possible.

Writing for your professional area

You can write up a research report for publication in a range of outlets including journals, books and other texts. Some journals accept more informal reports about new practices, while others require scholarly articles. Decide what is best for your purposes, and write according to the guidelines on the journal's website. It may sound over-ambitious to attempt to write for journal publication, but it is not. All publications come from real people like you: those people also do the shopping, sleep and everything else that people do. What makes them distinctive (and makes you distinctive if you try) is the courage and drive that makes them have a go, work at it and carry on until they succeed. If you have something important to say, say it and don't wait for someone else to say it for you. You have a right to research and write and speak for yourself, and a responsibility to do so. Throw anxieties to the winds and write.

Writing for the world

If you ever wanted to write a book, now is your chance. When you write you engage in a transformational process: you write what is in the head onto the page, which you then make public for the world. Key points here are:

- Be reasonably confident about what you wish to say and why you wish to say it. This may take time to work through. Talking with others can help you refine initial ideas and develop them into specific themes. Ask them for feedback as you write. Always give credit for their ideas and help.
- Stay on track. Don't wander off into interesting byways. Write out an initial action plan and stay with it. It can be helpful to produce an initial PowerPoint presentation for yourself, writing key ideas per slide in bullet point format. Keep this as your writing guide and add relevant ideas as they emerge.
- Be clear about who you are writing for. Identify your target audience – fellow nurses, policy makers or patient groups.
- Write in a style appropriate for your audience, and use language they are familiar with. Don't talk up or down to people; talk on the page as if you are talking to them face-to-face.

You can find massive amounts of advice on how to write for publication in books, articles and websites, and on the Internet.

Now consider the form of writing.

Form of writing

You can produce a range of texts, including the following.

Blogs, websites and social networking

This is probably the easiest and most accessible form of writing for communication. You can start a blog and use social media like Facebook, Twitter and email extensively. You can organise a potential global network to share ideas and learning surprisingly quickly. Web-based technology is improving all the time and it is not difficult to use, so there is no reason why you should not engage and enjoy the results.

Oral presentations

You can also do oral presentations when attending conferences or networked meetings. Follow the advice above about writing: keep to the point, be well prepared, and practise. Prepare for an oral presentation by rehearsing in your head, practising with a friend and talking to yourself in a mirror. Pack a bag of visual aids to use when doing your presentation. You do not need to do a PowerPoint presentation, but if you do, learn how to construct one and how to deliver ideas effectively. Again, plenty of advice on presentation techniques is available. Simple strategies include:

- Have confidence in yourself and your subject matter. If you believe in what you are saying, other people will pick up your enthusiasm and believe in it too.
- Aim for maximum participation and involvement. People respond to those who involve them in a conversation. Keep a light but serious touch throughout. Set up pair work or conversations in threes. Simply say, 'Ask the person next to you what they think'. It is wonderfully difficult to stop an audience of 100 people talking once they start.
- Talk in the language of the audience. If you are talking with nurses, use technical language if you wish. If you are talking with patients' families, use their language. Do not patronise. Keep everything simple and accessible. Do not assume that their unfamiliarity with technical language means they haven't an opinion. They do, and they will tell you if given the chance.
- Be prepared. Always organise your material in advance and be clear about what you are going to say and how you are going to say it. If you are nervous about presenting (who isn't?), play a video in your head of yourself presenting and act out the video.

Whatever you decide, be confident and enthusiastic and go for it. You would be amazed at what you can do that you didn't know you could until you try.

A final word about contributing to the public knowledge base.

5. CONTRIBUTING TO THE PUBLIC KNOWLEDGE BASE

A knowledge base contains all those texts – spoken, written or performed – that have ever been produced about a topic. Currently the knowledge base of nursing comprises mainly scholarly articles, books and policy statements written by people who have made their way into academic offices and boardrooms. Ironically, some of those people have worked little at bedsides but have gone straight into offices at officer level. Some are managerial or academic nurses who have learned how to manage systems with possibly little experience of the practical lifeworlds of patients. They often appear in the form of the academic and nursing elites that Schön (1983, 1995) spoke about; ironically they are allowed to present themselves as representing all nurses.

These are the people whose publications currently comprise the knowledge base. They are also the people who control what goes into it, because they are the reviewers and editors who make decisions about what gets published and therefore whose voices are heard and who is entitled to speak and be heard. It is another example of the circular structure of power (Dyrberg, 1997) that legitimises a system through its own legitimation processes.

This can change and should change, because it is damaging to clinical nurses and patients who need those in power to develop understanding about what their needs and hopes are. Patients need senior people and policy makers to have the experience of being a patient themselves, as Lord Mancroft did, reported on page 119. But things will not change unless someone actively makes them change: this is where you come in and make your contribution, though it brings risks and responsibilities. You need to decide to make your voice heard in the public domain through speaking and writing for publication. Putting your head above the parapet is risky because it means you will get shot at. This is where you make choices, because if you don't speak, no one will. It is no use looking for someone else because there is no one else. But the risk is worthwhile. You can contribute to a new knowledge base, comprising works produced by practitioners for practitioners, through producing your own account.

There is far to go, and nursing as a profession is already disadvantaged. Like some other professions, nursing has a history of elitism (Rafferty, 1996). This remains manifested in the social and organisational structures of nursing. These visible structures are rooted in the invisible epistemological structure, where abstract knowledge is more highly regarded than practical knowledge. This is where you can take action. You can actively work to transform the underlying abstract epistemology into a relational, inclusive epistemology, where all forms of knowledge and theory are valued and understood as contributing to new traditions of knowledge.

It takes courage and determination but this is what is needed to change the culture so that all nurses are seen as excellent practitioners and excellent theorists in their own right. The process starts here.

SUMMARY

This chapter has outlined what is involved in writing up your action research. It has explained the difference between validity and legitimacy, and emphasised the importance of establishing the legitimacy of your action research for different contexts and dimensions. Different forms of texts are described as well as the different audiences for whom they may be written. Advice is offered about developing good writing skills and habits. The need to make your work public becomes a special issue, for this is where you can find ways of influencing new directions for nursing and nursing research.

Reflective questions

- Can you articulate the importance of writing for publication? How does this give you and your action research legitimacy? Why is it essential?
- Can you say what is involved in writing a text for publication? Can you identify different audiences?
- What kind of writing skills and capacities are important? How do you develop them?
- Who will you write for? Why is it important to try to influence their thinking?
- How do you develop a self-perception of yourself as a writer as well as a researcher?

NINE

The significance of your action research

When you tell people about what you are doing in your action research, they often say, 'That sounds interesting but what's the point? So what?' This is an important question because it means you need to think about how your work is special, what you think it may achieve and why you need to communicate its importance to others.

This chapter discusses the importance of communicating the significance of your research to different groups, and how this operates in terms of the following dimensions: the personal (for yourself and your practice), the organisational (for your colleagues and for organisational practices), and the political (for your profession and for the wider world). We use the term 'dimension' as derived from Noffke (2009: 8) to communicate 'the multiple layers of assumptions, purposes and practices' involved. The chapter is therefore organised as follows:

1. The personal.
2. The professional.
3. The political.

These dimensions work as spheres of influence where you can encourage others also to explore their potentials for learning and in turn exercise their educational influence in the learning of others.

All are in a generative transformational relationship: the personal informs and transforms into the organisational, and this has implications for the political and wider processes of professional and social change. Also bear in mind that action research is an educational process that enables you to exercise your educational influence in your own and in other people's thinking.

Here are some ideas about the significance of your action research for the personal dimension, which includes your own learning and practice.

1. PERSONAL SIGNIFICANCE

All personal change begins in the mind. In a famous comment in relation to the peace process in Northern Ireland, when there was deep disagreement about the need for prior decommissioning by the IRA in order to reach agreement, John Hume, then leader of the SDLP observed that decommissioning begins in the mind rather than in the laying down of arms. We agree. Peace and any other initiative begin with the personal intent of the actor. You decide to take action to improve an unsatisfactory situation and you record the process of doing so.

This is especially important for clinical nurses in several respects, mainly in terms of demonstrating that they are competent practitioners and competent theorists. It does so in the following ways.

Demonstrating that you are a capable practitioner

Action and research take place in the practice area. By asking, 'How do I improve my practice as a nurse?' you show how you have developed your knowledge in terms of the following:

- factual information ('know-that') because you have studied substantive issues;
- procedural knowledge ('know-how') because you have developed skills and competencies;
- analytical and explanatory knowledge because you have linked know-that with know-how, and can say what you have done.

You have also developed communicative capacity because you can explicate the learning processes involved, and you can produce the evidence to test the validity of your claims that you have learnt, and now know at these different levels. This means you are actively taking responsibility for your practice and demonstrating accountability.

Because this research is based in the practice area and is practice led it follows that it is close to the patient. You may well have involved patients as co-researchers with other colleagues. This enhances a view of nursing as a dialogical, democratic practice developed in the field of action. It brings us closer to a situation where perfect health is not seen as a norm but as a guiding principle to influence ongoing real-life practices. It also helps us find ways of helping patients to exercise agency in their own flourishing rather than continuing the situation where patients feel they must hand their agency over to caring associations: the stories they tell contribute to a new knowledge base of nursing (see below).

In 1950s America a little boy was born with the hugely damaging and ultimately fatal condition of hydrocephalus, where fluid produced in the brain fails to drain, with resultant back-pressure. For some time doctors had experimented unsuccessfully with drainage systems but children continued to die. The father of the little boy was an engineer called John Holter who was not prepared to leave the matter to the doctors. On investigating, he found that the problem was a relatively simple engineering one which could be solved by creating a non-return valve. He developed this idea together with Dr Spitz of the medical staff. Although he eventually lost his son because of side effects of the condition, the Spitz-Holter valve came into being. It has, up to now, saved thousands of lives.

By making the patient the focus of enquiry you have reclaimed nursing as a caring practice and helped to re-establish the patient in the clinical area as the centre of gravity. By implication you have also re-established the legitimacy of the title 'nurse' for those who have demonstrated practical competence in caring for patients. A nurse is a person who works with patients in a demonstrably competent manner; the evidence base for your claim that you have done this is in patients' testimonies that they feel cared for and have been encouraged to engage more fully in their lives. This revisits the contested question: 'Who is a nurse?' Is 'nurse' only a protected title reserved for those who hold a paper qualification, or is it a term that refers to a person who nurses? Does 'nurse' mean a title or does it refer to a practice?

Demonstrating that you are a capable theorist

You have also created new learning for yourself and others and strengthened the link between knowledge and practice. By situating your action research in your own clinical workplace you have enabled practice to lead theory. This is hugely important because we talk so often about the theory–practice gap (see Rolfe, 1998), where established theory has little relevance for practice, whereas in fact the experience of many clinical nurses is that there is a practice–theory gap, in that continually developing practice often outpaces established theory.

You have extended your practice range by engaging in high-quality research and scholarship, and you can ground your claims to improved practices in a strong evidence base. By producing and explicating the process of producing an evidence base you show that you are a competent theorist. You also show yourself to be a scholar by engaging critically with the literatures. You can show how a focus on pragmatic issues has produced ongoing evidence of your professional development in the clinical situation, and you have gathered data and generated evidence to show the processes involved. You are now able to claim that you have extended your professionalism and professional range of responsibility by demonstrating how you have exercised your right to research, which Appadurai (2006) says is the responsibility of professionals. You have also demonstrated parrhesia by speaking for yourself, which Foucault (2001) identifies as a further responsibility. You have shown that you are qualified to engage in public discourses about what counts as valid nursing knowledge and about who is entitled to be seen as a knower.

Some years ago, nurses and doctors were disagreeing about how to care for dementia patients. The doctors, who paid brief visits to the wards and went by the received wisdom of the textbooks, said that the patients would just deteriorate regardless of the approach taken. The nurses, who knew the patients as individuals, insisted that encouraging the patients to do as much as possible for themselves could improve their quality of life. Although they did not call this research and considered it unethical to set up a control group which did not receive the same input, the nurses on one ward changed the way they treated patients. Whilst conversing with patients, the staff used the names of the patients' family members, talked about the here and now, encouraged them to dress themselves and comb their own hair, and look in mirrors and make choices about clothing. Although they did not attempt to do a comparative analysis, the doctors soon started to comment on the differences in mood, activity and levels of interaction between these dementia patients and other dementia patients on more traditional wards. This approach later came to be known as reality orientation. Looking back, the nurses can be criticised for not consulting the literatures. Perhaps their research method could have been more structured, but they achieved their main goal of making life better for their patients.

From these perspectives, you can appreciate how you are exercising your educational influence in your own thinking. You show that you are not content simply to go along with popular opinion or practice or internalise messages from the media. You can think for yourself as a person, claiming originality and willing to make your contribution with political intent. You can also exercise your educational influence in the thinking of others, including student nurses, to see the practice area as central to nursing theory, as we now explain.

2. PROFESSIONAL SIGNIFICANCE

The idea of exercising one's educational influence in the thinking of others is important. We believe that we are all born with the capacity to think for ourselves; it is part of our genetic inheritance as humans. This means that when we read advertisements or listen to public messages we can exercise our agency to block messages with which we disagree: we do not believe that men are from Mars and women are from Venus or that caring is something that women do rather than or better than men. We do not agree with the idea that patients are objects or a means to an end. As humans we choose to use our originality of mind to filter and critique whatever we are told so that we maintain our independence of thinking. We can then make appropriate judgements about our practices so that we are able to explain how we hold ourselves accountable for what we are doing.

The concept of education works from this principle. Education may be seen as a process whereby one person encourages another to learn how to exercise their independence of mind across all knowledge domains. Educators use their educational influence to enable others to think critically, but this involves appreciating that everyone can think for themselves. It also means that we can accept or reject the influence, and recognise it for what it is: the freedom to choose is honoured and maintained. As a thoughtful, caring nurse you do this: you try to exercise your educational influence in the thinking of others, as well as yourself. When other people share this or similar practices you form a community of practice. The challenge then is to turn communities of practice into communities of enquiry where all participants encourage others to engage in enquiry. A strong aspect of the significance of your research for the learning of others in your organisation or professional context is that you are able to do this.

By demonstrating these kinds of personal commitments and values, you can reclaim nursing both as an enquiring profession and as a caring profession: you show what it could mean for nursing to become an enquiring profession in the interests of others. The profession becomes centred around the needs of the client group (patients) so that the rational basis of nursing moves closer to its roots. It leads to patient-centred, health-centred cultures. Your research demonstrates how you and colleagues can build research-led evidence-based knowledge centred around your own practice.

This kind of research can be hugely beneficial for the profession as a whole. The decentralised and democratic nature of action research allows practitioners to take more of a leading role in knowledge development, and this can then lead to their having a stronger role in defining directions for the profession to take. This then decreases the danger of the profession being directed, as is currently the practice, by a narrow group whose focus is equally narrow regarding what kinds of knowledge qualify as important. It shows that, rather than being add-ons, practice-led approaches are core to defining a coherent, educational model of professionalism. This can bring nursing education and nursing research up to date with other professions that have already challenged narrow traditionalist approaches. These professions have replaced many of the old certainties with a more open-minded, questioning approach to the creation of knowledge, and developed this as the basis of professional practices.

However, this raises two important issues, to do with (1) the ownership of nursing research (and therefore what counts as nursing knowledge and theory), and consequently (2) who counts as a nurse and what qualifies nurses to enter the nursing profession.

3. POLITICAL SIGNIFICANCE

By engaging with these issues we have entered the realm of the political, which is by definition to do with power. Before engaging with broader issues, first consider how the idea of power is defined.

An interesting little book by Greene and Elferrs (1999) sets out 'the 48 Laws of Power'. These include:

- Conceal your intentions.
- Make other people come to you – use bait if necessary.
- Pose as a friend, work as a spy … and so on.

'Laws' such as these are symptomatic of a dominant form of discourse about power. Power is seen as a thing, a property that some people have and others do not. Theorists of this view of power include Dyrberg (1997) (as noted in this book) and Weber (1964). The aim of power struggles is to wrest power away from someone and claim it for oneself.

A different view of power is offered by Arendt (1958, 1973). Her view is that power is not a thing or a property of an individual, so much as people working together to achieve negotiated goals. This is when power happens – 'by coopera-tive effort between people who differ from one another yet have the capacity to come together' (Frazer, 2014: 156). The experience of engagement is dynamic and fluid: it takes the form of, to use Foucault's (1980a, 1980b) analogy, capil-lary action, when power permeates a system and finds its way into the smallest crevice of human being. We extend this view in this book to say that power takes the form of neural networks. The human brain is so constituted that it can process millions of bits of information in a split second. Further, this capacity is exponential: the more the brain computes, the greater its capacity for comput-ing becomes. Power works like this: the more people work together, the greater their strength. Nor is this capacity confined to clever or privileged people. The twenty-first century has become an era of capillary power in the form of social networks, greatly assisted by technology, where small groups of people have gen-erated worldwide movements, some for social good and others with a bent for destructive practices. Arendt believes that power is for the world and for 'the maintenance of "the in-between space" by which we are related to each other' (Frazer, 2014: 156). We agree, but we also maintain that it still comes down to people's intent: we can use those spaces for good or evil, for social good or social harm. Elites with an interest in self-preservation can come together as easily as democratically minded citizens. It is not an issue of whether or not people can come together; it is an issue of what they intend to do and how they intend to do it when they come together. Social networking can be used to encourage others to commit suicide just as easily as to eat sensibly.

Now consider the questions raised above, namely:

1. The ownership of nursing research (and therefore what counts as nursing knowledge and theory.
2. Who counts as a nurse and what qualifies nurses to enter the nursing profession.

The ownership of nursing research

We outlined in Chapter 2 that the purpose of research is to produce knowledge, which contributes to the generation of theory. The questions, 'Who is nursing knowledge and theory for?' and 'What is the purpose of nursing knowledge and theory?' are uncontested – nursing knowledge and theory are seen as for the benefit of the patients. What is in question, however, is (1) who says what counts as valid knowledge and therefore who owns the knowledge and the theory, and (2) who counts as a valid knower and therefore a theorist.

We said that currently the owners of nursing knowledge and nursing theory are academic nurses in universities and on professional bodies. Propositional knowledge and propositional theory, informed by commitments to technical rationality, are the most valued forms. Procedural knowledge is not valued in official terms, practical knowledge comes lower down, and personal knowledge has fallen off the page. Ironically (and a reminder of the words of Schön (1995)), procedural, practical and personal knowledge are all as essential to helping people get well as factual knowledge. This also has implications for who qualifies for entry to the profession.

What qualifies nurses to enter the nursing profession?

Currently, entry to nursing as a profession is by the narrow gateway of academic qualifications. School leavers need to achieve a certain number of high grades, working from a points system, to gain entry to universities, which is where nursing education is located. Some school leavers who dream of becoming a nurse find that they cannot fulfil their dreams because of lower grades or because there are insufficient places at university. Consequently, these bright young people who may be gifted in terms of practical skills and competencies but who lack academic qualifications are denied entry, and a whole swathe of talent is wasted. There is need for new professional pathways for such young people. The case is further strengthened by the fact that there will soon be a serious shortage of nurses in the UK. Already nurses are being drafted in from overseas to fill the staffing gaps. Why not create new pathways for eager young people to enter the profession with different routes to qualification, or different practice-based forms of qualification? Why not establish action research forms of training and practice, where people can develop professional pathways to different forms and levels of qualification, developed through studying practices?

Your research has demonstrated abundantly that researching one's practice in action can lead to enhanced forms of knowing, both conceptually and practically. Noffke (2009) says that action research itself may be seen as 'a distinctive way of knowing'. She says: 'This point is directly related to whether action research is seen as producing knowledge for others to use, or whether it is primarily as a means for professional development' (p. 10). She also says that 'action research has been seen as one way to enhance the professional quality and status of the profession' (p. 10). Noffke was speaking about the teaching profession: the same point relates equally to the nursing profession. It always returns to whether, in order to be a nurse, nurses need to have only specialist academic knowledge of the technical rational kind or also a more generalist humanistic-oriented form of embodied knowing that manifests as empathy and care. At the moment, we argue, nursing knowledge has been shoehorned into a narrow epistemological channel that can lead to disastrous outcomes for patients and families, as outlined earlier in this book, and which does egregious harm to the profession of nursing and those it serves.

Things do not have to be like this. When Habermas (1976) spoke about how humans create systems, he also made the point that they can recreate systems. If the systems we work with do not serve the purposes for which they were designed, they should change. This is the whole point of action research, where we find better ways of doing things and evaluate whether they work in practice and in theory. However, this brings implications for how we work, which is grounded in how we think. For, in order to recreate our systems, we also need to recreate the way we think, that is, reconceptualise what counts as nursing and especially what counts as nursing research. The main point here is to develop cultures of enquiry.

From communities of practice to communities of enquiry

We said above that it is important to recreate communities of practice as communities of enquiry. It is crucial to appreciate how each is distinctive.

A **community of practice** refers to a group of people who come together within the same practice domain, for a specific reason and with specific purposes. In nursing, senior and junior nurses come together, as do technicians, patients and families, and anyone else involved in the practice of nursing. The fact that they work together does not eliminate power relationships. Roles and responsibilities are maintained, frequently within hierarchically-organised systems. Discourses within communities often take the form of discussion and debate about substantive and procedural matters, such as treatments and procedures. Reasons and purposes may be diverse: people come together, for example, to find ways of raising the status of the profession or for the good of patients.

A **community of enquiry**, on the other hand, refers to a group of people who come together, not necessarily (although usually) in the same practice domain, specifically to find ways of improving their learning by engaging with others who are also learning. Enquiry is about learning. A community of enquiry is one whose focus is on learning, which also means research. As noted throughout, doing research means finding out something that you did not know already, or coming to know it better or differently, and deciding how to use your knowledge. In the case of communities of enquiry, the knowledge would always be used in terms of the community's interests. There is no guarantee that these interests would be for social good: they could equally be for harm. This is why it is important that, in nursing and other professions, we should aim to develop communities of educational enquiry, that is, communities whose focus is learning how to develop practices that are for the good of others, especially in terms of helping them to learn and to know better. While individuals may continue to have specific roles and responsibilities, hierarchical organisational power-constituted relationships would disappear since everyone would be learning with and from one another. It would be a community whose learning took the form of sharing mutually reciprocal beneficial knowledge, and with the capacity to explain how the knowledge was acquired and its potential significance for self and others. All would be involved: academic nurses, clinical nurses, patients, families – everyone in the community.

Developing a knowledge base for a community of educational enquiry

A community needs to build up its own knowledge base, comprising its spoken and written texts, to ground its knowledge claims. These texts provide a record to show how traditions develop within the community, and how the community can develop new traditions that reflect its values. In nursing, those texts would show the development of the traditions of patient-centred practices within an ethic of care and concern for the other; they would reflect the processes of internal reflection by individuals and groups that ensure that the practices recounted in the texts are not self-serving but aimed at the flourishing of the individual and the collective. The texts would be internally validated by the community, and made public for the external validation of others in the wider society.

This may sound visionary but it can be achieved. To demonstrate this, we would like to end this book with an update of a project that we feel privileged to be involved in.

We work with a group of Norwegian doctors and nurses, who are active in Cambodia and who have created a chain of survival for landmine victims by training medics in basic and advanced life support. Prior to their involvement, about 40% of the victims died before reaching hospital. Without proper treatment, many victims bled to death within the hour and others died on the way to hospital. The hospitals were located in the city; this meant hours of slow and costly transportation. The Norwegian team decided to build a 'chain of survival'. They developed an educational programme in basic and advanced life support for a core group of Cambodian medics. These medics in turn trained teams of local villagers to be first responders as injuries occurred in their immediate areas. Most of the villagers had no medical experience and some could not read or write. However, the team overcame the difficulties by developing simple, pragmatic training in the villages. Within a short time the chain of survival (village first responders and medics working together) was stopping blood loss, packing wounds, setting up intravenous fluids and accompanying victims to hospital. The mortality rate plummeted to 10% and the group then reset their sights on preserving limbs and function. The local volunteers then went on to train others and take a lead in deciding how to improve the service. Meanwhile, other non-governmental organisations maintained their view that locals cannot achieve this level of expertise and only qualified medical personnel are able to save lives and limbs. Further accounts of the work of the Norwegian team may be found in Husum (2000), Husum et al. (1995), Edvardsen (2006) and Houy et al. (2007).

New forms of practice and thinking are being achieved across the professions, including teaching and higher education. They can also be achieved in nursing. It does take time and effort but the potential benefits in terms of reclaiming nursing for nurses and patients are high. It is up to individual nurses to decide, including yourself.

SUMMARY

This chapter has discussed the importance of communicating the significance of your action research for different groupings and dimensions, including the personal, the professional and the political. In the personal dimension some of the main aspects of significance are that you show how you demonstrate that you are a capable practitioner and theorist. The professional dimension is where you are able to exercise your educational influence in the thinking of others, including those in your own organisation. The political significance is that you are able to contribute to public debates about who should own nursing knowledge, and the need for the development of nursing as a broad-based profession that includes and recognises all those involved in caring for patients. The chapter, like the entire book, encourages you to make your contribution to the knowledge base and values base of nursing for the good of the most important group – the patients.

References

Ah-See, K.W., Mackenzie, J., Thakker, N.S. and Maran, A.G.D. (1998) 'Local research ethics committee approval for a national study in Scotland', *Journal of the Royal College of Surgeons of Edinburgh*, 43(5): 303–305. Available at: www.rcsed.ac.uk/Journal/vol43_5/4350003.htm (accessed 29 July 2015).

Alford, C.F. (2001) *Whistleblowers: Broken Lives and Organizational Power*. Ithaca, NY: Cornell University Press.

Alligood, M.R. and Tomey, A.M. (eds) (2010) *Nursing Theorists and Their Work* (7th edn). Maryland Heights, MO: Mosby Elsevier.

al-Takriti, N. (2010) 'Negligent mnemocide and the shattering of Iraqi collective Memory', in R. Baker, S. Ismael and T. Ismael (eds), *Cultural Cleansing in Iraq*. London: Pluto Press, pp. 93–115.

Antonovsky, A. (1979) *Health, Stress and Coping*. San Francisco, CA: Jossey-Bass.

Appadurai, A. (2006) 'The right to research', *Globalizations, Societies and Education*, 4(2): 167–177.

Arendt, H. (1958) *The Human Condition*. Chicago, IL: University of Chicago Press.

Arendt, J. (1968) *Men in Dark Times*. San Diego, CA: Harcourt Brace & Co.

Arendt H. (1973) *On Revolution*. London: Pelican.

Bakhtin, M. (1986) *The Dialogical Imagination* (ed. M. Holquist). Austin, TX: University of Texas Press.

Barrett, J. and Whitehead, J. (1985) 'Supporting teachers in their classroom research'. Working paper, Bath, University of Bath, School of Education.

Bell, J. (2005) *Doing Your Research Project* (4th edn). Maidenhead: Open University Press.

Bellman, L. (2012) 'Ethical Considerations' in G.R. Williamson, L. Bellman and J. Webster (eds), *Action Research in Nursing and Healthcare*. Thousand Oaks, CA: Sage, pp. 146–166.

Benner, P. (1984) *From Novice to Expert: Excellence and Power in Clinical Nursing Practice*. Menlo Park, CA: Addison-Wesley.

Benner, P., Sutphen, M., Leonard, V. and Day, L. (2010) *Educating Nurses: A Call for Radical Transformation*. San Francisco, CA: Jossey-Bass.

Benner, P., Tanner, C. and Chesla, C. (1996) *Expertise in Nursing Practice: Caring, Clinical Judgment, and Ethics*. New York: Springer.

Bereiter, C. and Scardamalia, M. (1987) *The Psychology of Written Composition*. Hillsdale, NJ: Lawrence Erlbaum Associates.

Berlin, I. (1990) *The Crooked Timber of Humanity: Chapters in the History of Ideas* (ed. H. Hardy). London: Chatto & Windus.

Berwick, D. (2013) Bewick Review into Patient Safety: *A Promise to Learn – A Commitment to Act. National Advisory Group on the Safety of Patients in England.* London, Department of Health. Available at: https://www.gov.uk/government/uploads/system/uploads/attachment_data/file/226703/Berwick_Report.pdf (accessed 29 July 2015)

Binnie, A. and Titchen, A. (1999) *Freedom to Practise.* Oxford: Butterworth-Heinemann.

Bohm, D. (1996) *On Dialogue* (ed. L. Nichol). London: Routledge.

Bohman, J. and Lutz-Bachmann, M. (1997) *Perpetual Peace: Essays on Kant's Cosmopolitan Ideal.* Cambridge, MA: MIT Press.

Bourdieu, P. (1990) *The Logic of Practice.* Cambridge: Polity.

Boyer, E. (1990) *Scholarship Reconsidered: Priorities of the Professoriate.* Princeton, NJ: Carnegie Foundation for the Advancement of Teaching.

British Educational Research Association (2011) *Ethical Guidelines.* Available at: https://www.bera.ac.uk/researchers-resources/publications/ethical-guidelines-for-educational-research-2011 (accessed 26 February 2015).

Brookfield, S. (1987) *Developing Critical Thinkers.* Milton Keynes: Open University Press.

Buber, M. (1937) *I and Thou* (trans. R.G. Smith). Edinburgh: Clark.

Buber, M. (2002) *Between Man and Man.* London: Routledge.

Burnard, P., Morrison, P. and Gluyas, H. (2011) *Nursing Research in Action* (3rd edn). Houndmills, Basingstoke: Palgrave Macmillan.

Butler-Kisber, L. (2010) *Qualitative Inquiry.* London: Sage.

Campbell, A. and Groundwater-Smith, S. (eds) (2007) *An Ethical Approach to Practitioner Research.* Abingdon: Routledge.

Carr, W. and Kemmis, S. (1986) *Becoming Critical: Education, Knowledge and Action Research.* London: Falmer.

Chomsky, N. (1986) *Knowledge of Language: Its Nature, Origin and Use.* New York: Praeger.

Chomsky, N. (1997) *Media Control: The Spectacular Achievements of Propaganda.* New York: Seven Stories Press.

Coghlan, D. and Brannick, T. (2001) *Doing Action Research in Your Own Organization.* London: Sage.

Cranmer, P. and Nhemachena, J. (2013) *Ethics for Nurses: Theory and Practice.* Maidenhead: Open University Press.

Creswell, J. (2007) *Qualitative Inquiry and Research Design* (2nd edn). Thousand Oaks, CA: Sage.

Cummings, J. (2012) *Compassion in Practice: Nursing, Midwifery and Care Staff. Our Vision and Strategy.* London: Department of Health. Available at: www.england.nhs.uk/wp-content/uploads/2012/12/compassion-in-practice.pdf (accessed 20 May 2013).

Cuthbert, S. and Quallington, J. (2008) *Values for Care Practice.* Exeter: Reflect Press.

Czikszentmihalyi, M. (1990) *Flow.* New York: HarperPerennial.

Denzin, N.K. (1989) *The Research Act* (3rd edn). London: Prentice Hall.

Department of Health (2012) *Caring for Our Future: Reforming Care and Support.* London: DH. Available at: www.gov.uk/government/publications/caring-for-our-future-reforming-care-and-support (accessed 29 July 2015).

Derrida, J. (1976) *Of Grammatology.* Baltimore, MD: Johns Hopkins University Press.

Dewey, J. (1963) *Experience and Education.* New York: Collier Books.

Dunne, J. (1997) *Back to the Rough Ground.* Notre Dame, IN: University of Notre Dame Press.

Dyrberg, T. (1997) *The Circular Structure of Power.* London: Verso.

Edvardsen, O. (2006) 'A network for first aid in the mine-infested area of North Iraq'. Masters dissertation, Tromsø, University of Tromsø.

Eikeland, O. (2011) 'Condescending ethics and action research', *Action Research*, 4(1): 37–47.

Elliott, J. (1991) *Action Research for Educational Change*. Maidenhead: Open University Press.

Elliott, J. (2003) 'The struggle to redefine the relationship between "knowledge" and "action" in the academy: Some reflections on action research'. Available at: www.uab.cat/web?blobcol=urldocument&blobheader=application%2Fpdf&blobkey=id&blobnocache=true&blobtable=Document&blobwhere=1096479622851&ssbinary=true (accessed 29 July 2015).

Eraut, M. (1994) *Developing Professional Knowledge and Competence*. London: Falmer.

Flood, R.L. (2001) 'The relationship of "systems thinking" to action research', in P. Reason and H. Bradbury (eds), *Handbook of Action Research: Participative Inquiry & Practice*. London: Sage, pp. 133–144.

Foucault, M. (1980a) 'Questions of method', in J.D. Faubion (ed.), *Michel Foucault: Power* (Vol. 3). New York: The New Press, pp. 223–238.

Foucault, M. (1980b) 'Truth and power' in C. Gordon (ed.), *Power/Knowledge: Selected Interviews and Other Writings, 1972–1977*. Brighton: Harvester.

Foucault, M. (2001) *Fearless Speech*. Los Angeles, CA: Semiotext(e).

Francis, R. (2013) *Report of the Mid-Staffordshire NHS Foundation Trust Public Inquiry*. London: The Stationery Office.

Francis, R. (2015) *Freedom to Speak Up. An Independent Review into Creating an Open and Honest Reporting Culture in the NHS*. Available at: https://freedomtospeakup.org.uk/wp-content/uploads/2014/07/F2SU_web.pdf (accessed 29 July 2015).

Frankl, V. (1959) *Man's Search for Meaning*. Boston, MA: Beacon.

Frazer, E. (2014) 'Power and violence', in P. Hayden (ed.), *Hannah Arendt: Key Concepts*. Durham: Acumen Press, pp. 155–166.

Freire, P. (1970) *Pedagogy of the Oppressed*. New York: Herder and Herder.

Freshwater, D. and Rolfe, G. (2004) *Deconstructing Evidence-Based Practice*. Abingdon, Oxon: Routledge.

Fromm, E. (1956) *The Art of Loving*. New York: Harper and Row.

Fry, K. (2014) 'Natality' in P. Hayden (ed.), *Hannah Arendt: Key Concepts*. Durham: Acumen Publishing, pp. 23–35.

Ghaye, T. and Lillyman, S. (2010) *Reflection: Principles and Practices for Healthcare Professionals* (2nd edn). London: Quay Books.

Gibbons, M., Limoges, C., Nowotny, H., Schwartzman, S., Scott, P. and Trow, M. (1994) *The New Production of Knowledge: The Dynamics of Science and Research in Contemporary Societies*. London: Sage.

Gray, J. (1995) *Enlightenment's Wake: Politics and Culture and the Close of the Modern Age*. London, Routledge.

Greene, R. and Elffers, J. (1999) *Power: The 48 Laws* (concise edition). London: Profile Books.

Greenwood, D. and Levin, M. (2007) *Introduction to Action Research* (2nd edn). Thousand Oaks, CA: Sage.

Habermas, J. (1972) *Knowledge and Human Interests* (trans. J.J. Shapiro). London: Heinemann.

Habermas, J. (1975) *Legitimation Crisis*. Boston, MA: Beacon Press.

Habermas, J. (1976) *Communication and the Evolution of Society*. Boston, MA: Beacon.

Hammersley, M. and Traianou, A. (2012) *Ethics and Educational Research*. British Educational Research Association online resource. Available at: https://www.bera.ac.uk/wp-content/uploads/2014/02/Ethics-and-Educational-Research.pdf (accessed 26 February 2015).

Hansard, Lord (2008) *Parliamentary Business, Publications and Records*. 28 February: Column 825 (London). Available at: www.publications.parliament.uk/pa/ld200708/ldhansrd/text/80228-0011.htm (accessed 15 June 2015).

Hart, E. and Bond, M. (1995) *Action Research for Health and Social Care*. Buckingham: Open University Press.

Higgs, J. and Titchen, A. (2001) *Practice Knowledge and Expertise in the Health Professions*. Oxford: Butterworth Heinemann.

Higgs, J., Titchen, A., Horsfall, D. and Bridges, D. (2011) *Creating Spaces for Qualitative Researching*. Rotterdam: Sense Publishers.

Herr, K. and Anderson, G. (2005) *The Action Research Dissertation*. New York: Sage.

Houy, C., Steinholt, M. and Husum, H. (2007) 'Delivery life support: A preliminary report on the chain of survival for complicated deliveries in rural Cambodia', *Nursing and Health Sciences*, 9(4): 263–269.

Hume, D. (1985) *A Treatise of Human Nature*. London: Penguin Classics.

Husum, H. (2000) *Save Lives, Save Limbs: Life Support for Victims of Mines, Wars and Accidents*. Penang: Third World Network.

Husum, H., Swee Chai Ang and Fosse, E. (1995) *War Surgery: Field Manual*. Penang: Third World Network.

Jacobs, G. (2006) 'Imagining the flowers, but working the rich and heavy clay: participation and empowerment in action research for health', *Educational Action Research*, 14(4): 569–581.

Johnson, J. and Ratner, P. (1997) 'The nature of knowledge used in nursing practice', in S.E. Thorne and V.E. Hayes (eds), *Nursing Praxis: Knowledge and Action*. Thousand Oaks, CA: Sage, pp. 3–22.

Kuhn, T. (1996) *The Structure of Scientific Revolutions* (3rd edn). London: University of Chicago Press.

Lave, J. and Wenger, E. (1991) *Situated Learning: Legitimate Peripheral Participation*. Cambridge: Cambridge University Press.

Laws, S. with Harper, C. and Marcus, R. (2003) *Research for Development*. London: Sage Publications.

Lewin, K. (1946) 'Action research and minority problems', *Journal of Social Issues*, 2(4): 34–46.

Liaschenko, J. (1997) 'Knowing the patient?', in S.E. Thorne and V.E. Hayes (eds), *Nursing Praxis: Knowledge and Action*. Thousand Oaks, CA: Sage.

Lyotard, J.-F. (1984) *The Postmodern Condition: A Report on Knowledge*. Manchester: Manchester University Press.

Macmurray, J. (1957) *The Self as Agent*. London: Faber and Faber.

Macmurray, J. (1961) *Persons in Relation*. London: Faber and Faber.

Marx, K. (1987) *The Eighteenth Brumaire of Louis Bonaparte*. New York: International Publishers.

Mason, J. (2002) *Qualitative Researching* (2nd edn). London: Sage.

McCormack, B. and McCance, T. (2010) *Person-Centred Nursing: Theory and Practice*. Oxford: Blackwell.

McDonnell, P. and McNiff, J. (2013) *Action Research for Professional Selling*. Farnham: Gower.

McNamee, M. (2002) 'Introduction: Whose Ethics, Which Research?', in M. McNamee and D. Bridges (eds), *The Ethics of Educational Research*. Oxford: Blackwell.

McNiff, J. (1984) 'Action research: A generative model for in-service education', *British Journal of Education*, 10(3): 40–46.

McNiff, J. (2010) *Action Research for Professional Development*. Poole: September Books.

McNiff, J. (2013) *Action Research: Principles and Practice* (3rd edn). Abingdon: Routledge.

McNiff, J. (2014) *Writing and Doing Action Research*. London: Sage.

McNiff, J. (2015) *Writing Up Your Action Research Project*. Abingdon: Routledge.

McNiff, J. (2016, in preparation) *You and Your Action Research Project* (4th edn). Abingdon: Routledge.

Melnyk, B.M. and Fineout-Overholt, E. (2005) *Evidence-Based Practice in Nursing and Healthcare*. Philadelphia, PA: Lippincott, Williams & Wilkins.

Mendieta, E. (2006) 'Introduction', in R. Rorty, *Take Care of Freedom and Truth Will Take Care of Itself: Interviews with Richard Rorty* (ed. D. Mendieta). Stanford, CA: Stanford University Press.

Meyer, J. (2006) 'Becoming connected, being caring', *Educational Action Research*, 14(4): 477–496.

Mezirow, J. (2009) 'An overview on transformative learning', in K. Illeris (ed.), *Contemporary Theories of Learning*. Abingdon: Routledge. pp. 90–105.

Midgley, J. (2008) Perspectives on globalization and culture: Implications for social work practices, *Journal of Global Social Work Practice*, 1(1): 1–11.

Mouffe, C. (2013) *Agonistics: Thinking the World Politically*. London: Verso.

Moule, P. and Hek, G. (2011) *Making Sense of Research* (4th edn). London: Sage.

Noddings, N. (1984) *Caring: A Feminine Approach to Ethics and Moral Education*. Berkeley, CA: University of California Press.

Noffke, S. (2009) 'Revisiting the professional, personal, and political dimensions of action research', in S. Noffke and B. Somekh (eds), *The SAGE Handbook of Educational Action Research*. London: Sage, pp. 6–23.

Nursing and Midwifery Council (2015) *The Code: Professional Standards of Practice and Behaviour for Nurses and Midwives*. London: NMC. Available at: www.nmc.org.uk/global assets/sitedocuments/nmc-publications/revised-new-nmc-code.pdf (accessed 29 July 2015).

O'Reilly, P. (1984) *Writing for the Market*. Dublin: Mercier Press.

Parlett, M. and Hamilton, D. (eds) (1977) *Beyond the Numbers Game*. Basingstoke: Macmillan.

Peate, I. and Nair, M. (eds) (2011) *Fundamentals of Anatomy and Physiology for Student Nurses*. Oxford: Blackwell.

Polanyi, M. (1958) *Personal Knowledge*. London: Routledge & Kegan Paul.

Polanyi, M. (1983) *The Tacit Dimension*. Gloucester, MA: Peter Smith.

Quallington, J. and Perry, J. (2014) 'Patient-centred research: A new approach to care', *Practice Nursing*, 25(2): 94–97.

Rafferty, A. (1996) *The Politics of Nursing Knowledge*. London: Routledge.

Rawls, J. (1972) *A Theory of Justice*. Oxford: Oxford University Press.

Reason, P. and Bradbury, H. (2008) 'Introduction', in P. Reason and H. Bradbury (eds), *The SAGE Handbook of Action Research* (2nd edn). London: Sage, pp. 1–13.

Reason, P. and Rowan, J. (1981) *Human Inquiry: A Sourcebook for New Paradigm Research*. London: Wiley.

Reid-Searl, K., Dwyer, T., Ryan, J., Moxham, L. and Richards, A. (2012) *Clinical Skills* (2nd edn). Harlow: Pearson.

Rolfe, G. (1996) *Closing the Theory-Practice Gap*. Oxford: Butterworth Heinemann.

Rolfe, G. (1998) *Expanding Nursing Knowledge*. Oxford: Butterworth Heinemann.

Rolfe, G. (2006) 'Evidence-based practice', in M. Jasper, *Professional Development, Reflection and Decision-Making*. Oxford: Blackwell, pp. 135–153.

Rorty, R. (2006) *Take Care of Freedom and Truth will Take Care of Itself: Interviews with Richard Rorty* (ed. D. Mendieta). Stanford, CA: Stanford University Press.

Royal College of Nursing (2005) *Maxi Nurses: Nurses Working in Advanced and Extended Roles Promoting and Developing Patient-Centred Health Care*. London: Royal College of Nursing. Available at: www.rcn.org.uk/__data/assets/pdf_file/0004/78646/002511.pdf (accessed 29 July 2015).

Royal College of Nursing (2012) *Advanced Nurse Practitioners: An RCN Guide to Advanced Nursing Practice, Advanced Nurse Practitioners and Programme Accreditation*. London: Royal College of Nursing. Available at: www.rcn.org.uk/__data/assets/pdf_file/0003/146478/003207.pdf (accessed 29 July 2015).

Ryle, G. (1949) *The Concept of Mind*. Chicago: University of Chicago Press.

Said, E. (1994) *Representations of the Intellectual: The 1993 Reith Lectures*. London: Vintage.

Schön, D. (1983) *The Reflective Practitioner: How Professionals Think in Action*. New York: Basic Books.

Schön, D. (1995) 'Knowing-in-action: The New Scholarship requires a new epistemology', *Change*, November–December: 27–32.

Schön, D. and Rein, M. (1994) *Frame Reflection*. New York: Basic Books.

Secretary of State for Health & Secretary of State for the Home Department (2003) *The Victoria Climbié Inquiry: A Report by Lord Laming*. London, January 2003 (CM.5730).

Seely Brown, J. and Duguid, P. (2000) *The Social Life of Information*. Boston, MA: Harvard Business School Press.

Seligman, M. (2011) *Flourish*. London: Nicholas Brealey.

Senge, P., Scharmer, C.O., Jaworski, J. and Flowers, B.S. (2005) *Presence: Exploring Profound Change in People, Organizations and Society*. London: Nicholas Brealey Publishing.

Sennett, R. (2008) *The Craftsman*. London: Penguin.

Sharples, M. (1999) *How We Write*. London: Routledge.

Stenhouse, L. (1983) 'Research is systematic enquiry made public', in *British Educational Research Journal*, 9(1): 11–20.

Sternberg, R. and Horvath, J. (1999) *Tacit Knowledge in Professional Practice*. Mahwah, NJ: Lawrence Erlbaum Associates.

Streubert Speziale, H.J. and Carpenter, D.R. (2007) *Qualitative Research in Nursing: Advancing the Human Imperative*. London: Lippincott Williams and Wilkins.

Stringer, E. (2007) *Action Research* (3rd edn). Thousand Oaks, CA: Sage.

Sumara, D. and Davis, B. (2009) 'Complexity theory and action research', in S. Noffke and B. Somekh (eds), *Handbook of Educational Action Research*. London: Sage, pp. 358–369.

Taylor, B. (2000) *Reflective Practice: A Guide for Nurses and Midwives*. Maidenhead: Open University Press.

Tharp, T. (2006) *The Creative Habit: Learn it and Use it For Life*. New York: Simon & Schuster.

The King's Fund (2013) *Patient-Centred Leadership: Rediscovering Our Purpose*. London: The King's Fund.

The Telegraph (2012) 'My husband died because people didn't care', 5 December 2012. Available at: www.telegraph.co.uk/news/health/9724205/Ann-Clwyd-My-husband-died-because-people-didnt-care.html#article (accessed 27 February 2015).

Thorne, S. and Hayes, V. (eds) (1997) *Nursing Praxis: Knowledge and Action*. Thousand Oaks, CA: Sage.

Titchen, A. and Ersser, S. (2001) 'Explicating, creating and validating professional craft knowledge', in J. Higgs and A. Titchen (2001) *Practice Knowledge and Expertise*. Oxford: Butterworth Heinemann, pp. 48–56.

Torbert, W. (2001) 'The practice of action inquiry', in P. Reason and H. Bradbury (eds), *Handbook of Action Research*. London: Sage, pp. 250–260.

Torbert, W.R. and Taylor, S.T. (2008) 'Action inquiry: Interweaving multiple qualities', in P. Reason and H. Bradbury (eds), *The SAGE Handbook of Action Research* (2nd edn). London: Sage, pp. 239–251.

Tovey, E. and Adams, A. (2001) 'The changing nature of nurses' job satisfaction: An exploration of sources of satisfaction in the 1990s', *Journal of Advanced Nursing*, 30(1): 150–158.

Triggle, N. (2013) Prime Minister Cameron defends plans for nursing shake-up. Available at: www.bbc.co.uk/news/health-22209634 (accessed 20 May 2013).

Von Dietz, E. and Orb, A. (2000) 'Compassionate care: A moral dimension of nursing', *Nursing Inquiry*, 7(3): 166–174.

Vuthy, S., Nath, C., Chandy, H., Sano, R., Edvardsen, O. and Ingstad, B. (2014) 'Disabled people community workshop: A qualitative study about the use and effects of the workshop run by local landmine amputees in Samlot district, Battambang', in Trauma Care Foundation *Results of Medical Research Course*. Tromsø and Battambang: Trauma Care Foundation.

Weber, M. (1964) *The Theory of Social and Economic Organization* (ed. T. Parsons). New York: The Free Press.

Wenger, E. (1998) *Communities of Practice: Learning, Meaning and Identity*. Cambridge: Cambridge University Press.

Whitehead, J. (1989) 'Creating a living educational theory from questions of the kind, "How do I improve my practice?"', *Cambridge Journal of Education*, 19(1): 137–153.

Williamson, G., Bellman, L. and Webster, J. (2012) *Action Research in Nursing and Healthcare*. London: Sage.

Winter, R. and Munn-Giddings, C. (2001) *A Handbook for Action Research in Health and Social Care*. London: Routledge.

Yin, R. (2009) *Case Study Research: Design and Methods* (4th edn). Thousand Oaks, CA: Sage.

Zeni, J. (2001) (ed.) *Ethical Issues in Practitioner Research*. New York: Teachers College Press.

Index